SHARED CARE OF **Older People**

Commissioning Editor: Alison Taylor
Development Editor: Catherine Jackson
Project Manager: Nancy Arnott
Designer: Stewart Larking
Illustration Manager: Bruce Hogarth

Preface

This book aims to provide a concise and practical guide to help understanding of the most common and important areas of medicine of old age. The authors are two specialists in medicine of old age and two general practitioners. We all have experience of the everyday challenges of providing health care to older people and are actively involved in both undergraduate and postgraduate teaching. What we offer is a set of self-contained, 'bite-sized' chapters that can be read in order, or more likely dipped into at different stages. Each of the chapters could be used for reference when dealing with a particular patient's problems or as the basis of a tutorial. All will be helpful in preparing for GP Summative Assessment and the MRCGP or the Diploma in Geriatric Medicine offered by the Royal College of Physicians.

Through the use of brief case studies each chapter covers the essential aspects of diagnosis and management of the major conditions that all primary care professionals will commonly encounter within any ageing population. Emphasis is placed throughout on integrated and practical clinical management in the community by the primary care team and appropriate sharing of care with hospital specialists.

We hope the book will address the needs especially of general practitioners and community and practice nurses in training, but also provide a useful reference for other more or less experienced health and social care professionals working together in the expanding field of elderly care. The approach we have taken aims to add clinical relevance to current policies designed to improve health in later life, particularly the National Service Framework for Older People and the Chronic Disease

Management programme. The practical emphasis of the book should also appeal to medical and nursing undergraduates, all of whom study medicine of old age and elderly care as part of their core curriculum.

We are grateful to our colleagues and students who have read and commented on the material contained within these pages. Thanks also must go to Heidi Harrison, Robert Edwards, Catherine Jackson and Alison Taylor of Elsevier Ltd, all of whom have helped to steer the book through to publication.

Gurcharan Rai
Joe Rosenthal
Jackie Morris
Steve Iliffe

London 2006

Foreword

In their introduction to this book Gurcharan Rai and his colleagues quite rightly state that medical care in Great Britain is changing. Organisational changes abound. New arrangements for commissioning and providing services seem to be announced continuously, with ever increasing increases in the pace of change. One area that has been rather slower to change has been the division between services provided by general practitioners (primary care) and hospitals (secondary care). However in this area too, things are developing. Consultant geriatrician posts are being created with responsibility for linking with primary care, whilst General Practitioners with a specialist interest in older people are being recognised and rewarded as such. It is interesting to reflect that in the USA, one's competency as a geriatrician can be certified after first training in either family medicine or in general (internal) medicine. Perhaps this might also happen in the UK.

Defining the respective roles and responsibilities of the primary and secondary health care sectors in the diagnosis and management of medical conditions, is now accepted as an essential part of any clinical guideline. This principle is being now being extended to the management of both acute and chronic conditions affecting older people and this volume complements this process.

This book will be of value as an introductory text to both doctors and allied health professionals working in primary care and in hospital. The expert authors have produced a text which uses a lively, imaginative approach using case histories that illustrate the common clinical problems in later life. Thus it will also provide an excellent start for a student tutorial. I can thoroughly recommend this book for trainers and trainees to raise awareness and confidence in providing improved treatments to older people.

Peter Crome MD PhD FRCP FFPM
President-Elect, British Geriatrics Society
Professor of Geriatric Medicine

Keele University Medical School
Staffordshire
August 2005

Content

CHAPTER 1

Caring for older people in primary care

Introduction

Medical care in Great Britain is about to change. Those now entering general practice and many specialist disciplines—but particularly medicine for the elderly—will work through the greatest transformation in service provision since the foundation of the NHS in 1948. One part of that change will be in the decentralisation of responsibilities for organising services, with a corresponding increase in regulation and inspection to ensure that responsibilities are discharged. Another part, which in a sense is the subject of this book, will be the blurring of boundaries between generalists and specialists, between primary and secondary care. In the following chapters we discuss the 'shared care' of patients with different kinds of clinical problems, as an administrative and organisational way of re-distributing knowledge and skills between specialists and generalists. From shared care it is only a few steps to joint clinical directorates and a common clinical governance framework, applied to medical care in the community and in hospital. The structure of medical practice will be re-engineered to create a more efficient and effective division of labour between disciplines, training will become aligned to disease management rather than professional category and primary and secondary care clinicians will work together to design and deliver effective care management.

This process of change is one in which we have ample time to experiment, innovate and learn from experience, although those enduring a flurry of initiatives and directives from the Department of Health and the NHS Executive might feel that there is some urgency about adapting to an ageing society. There is not. As we have argued before, our society is not ageing rapidly (Iliffe et al 1998). Since 1981 there has been no increase in the proportion of the population aged 65 and over, currently standing at around 16% of the total population. This age group will probably rise to 17% by 2011 (Arber 1996). Those aged 85 or more will constitute 12% of the older population (defined as those aged 65 or more) but only 1% of the total population. It is this increase that makes health service planners anxious, since a large part of disability is found in this population group, and individuals can have complex and multiple disease processes requiring frequent contact with services.

However, we do not need to panic about this change, for we are living through a pause in the process of demographic ageing and probably face only a modest increase in the size of the older population in the first quarter of the 21st century, with a projected increase amongst those aged 60 and over from 20% to 24% (Warnes 1989). Sweden experienced such a change in the middle of the 20th century, and became one of the most stable and successful societies in Europe. Projected increases in the proportion of older people in the population at the beginning of this century are neither new nor unprecedented, and they will be significantly less than increases in under-developed countries, which will experience the greatest problems of service provision. Anxieties about the ageing of the British population and the effect of demography on provision of health and social services are, therefore, less to do with the absolute numbers of older people than to do with heightened expectations about the type, length and costs of such care.

We are unlikely to run out of resources because of demographic ageing, although if the NHS continues to treat its staff badly we may well experience an unavoidable exodus alongside a failure to recruit. Older people in Britain in the 21st century will have more resources than any equivalent population has had before. Changing marriage and fertility patterns over the last 50 years have resulted in the expansion of the social networks of older people. In 1977, one-third of those aged

75 or over had no children, but by the early 1990s this had fallen to nearer 16%. More is demanded of older people by their children and grandchildren, and more support is offered to them, contrary to the myth that children neglect and abandon their ageing parents. The result is that older people provide over a third of the so-called informal care of ill and disabled individuals, act as a major source of childcare for the increasing proportion of working mothers and provide the backbone of voluntary support in the health service and in voluntary organisations that contribute on a broad scale to health and social care.

Even concerns about the impact of disability in the oldest old could turn out to be exaggerated. Instead of the pandemic of disability and dementia implied in apocalyptic interpretations of demographic change, most of the gain in life expectancy seems to be occurring without disability (Robine & Ritchie 1991). A woman of 65 with 17.6 years life expectancy will remain fit and active for 9 or 10 years, and a man of the same age, with a life expectancy of 13.7 years, for 7 or 8 years. American studies of cohorts of older people during the 1980s showed that the decline in disabling conditions was most pronounced for disorders of the heart and circulation (Manton et al 1995). In these studies the probability that a person aged 85 or over remained free of disabilities increased by nearly 30% during the 1980s. This is not to say that Fries's theory about the compression of morbidity into the last few months of life (Fries 1980) (with an active, fit existence suddenly turning into disability and fatal illness over a short period of time) has been proved true for the whole population. A very significant minority of older people do have major, disabling problems that require medical, nursing and social support if anything like normal life is to be maintained, and the prevalence of major neurological and musculoskeletal causes of disability (e.g.

stroke, the dementias, Parkinson's disease, osteoarthritis and fractured neck of femur) is likely to rise (Tallis 1992). This is why we do need to re-configure our care for older people, and acquire new clinical and organisational skills.

The processes of re-engineering are underway, but will take time to become dominant within the culture of either hospital medicine or general practice. There are two important precursors to the major changes that we are describing, which will promote and shape shared care for older people. They are the National Service Framework for Older People (DoH 2001), and the chronic disease management (CDM) programme. We will summarise each in turn.

The National Service Framework for Older People

The National Service Framework for Older People (NSFOP) is the key implementation guidance for health and social care services. It is a comprehensive strategy to ensure fair, high-quality, integrated health and social care services for older people and outlines a 10-year programme of action. It links services to support independence and promote health, specialised services for key conditions and a cultural change fostering treatment of older people and their carers with respect, dignity and fairness.

Throughout the document older people are regarded as a heterogeneous group, with particular emphasis on the needs of ethnic elders, and it advocates that all services reflect the diversity of the population they serve, including the needs of carers. Addressing ageism in public services is seen as an integral component of the modernisation of health and social care services, and rooting out age discrimination is the first standard in the NSFOP.

The NSFOP focuses on four key themes with the eight standards flowing through them. The standards address conditions particularly significant for older people that are not covered in other National Service Frameworks: stroke, falls and mental health problems associated with old age. The themes and standards are shown in Box 1.1.

BOX 1.1: NSFOP themes and standards

Theme 1: Respecting the individual
Standard 1: Rooting out age discrimination. NHS services will be provided, regardless of age, on the basis of clinical need alone. Social care services will not use age in their eligibility criteria or policies, to restrict access to available services.

Standard 2: Person-centred care. NHS and social care services should treat older people as individuals and enable them to make choices about their own care, achieved through: the single assessment process; integrated commissioning arrangements; integrated service provision, including community equipment and continence services.

Theme 2: Intermediate care
Standard 3: Intermediate care. Older people will have access to a new range of intermediate care services at home or designated care settings, to promote their independence by providing NHS and LA services to prevent unnecessary hospital admission, and rehabilitation services to enable early hospital discharge and prevent admission to long-term residential care.

Theme 3: Providing evidenced-based specialist care
Standard 4: General hospital care. Older people's care in hospital is delivered through appropriate specialist care and by hospital staffs that have the right sets of skills to meet their needs.

BOX 1.1: NSFOP themes and standards—continued

Standard 5: Stroke. The NHS will take action to prevent strokes, working in partnership with other agencies where appropriate. People diagnosed with having had a stroke are managed by a specialist stroke service, and with their carers, participate in a multidisciplinary programme of secondary prevention and rehabilitation.

Standard 6: Falls. The NHS, working in partnership with councils, acts to prevent falls and reduce resultant injuries in older people. Older people who have fallen receive treatment and rehabilitation and, with their carers, receive advice on prevention through a specialist falls service.

Standard 7: Mental health services. Older people who have mental health problems can access integrated mental health services, provided by the NHS and councils to ensure effective diagnosis, treatment and support, for them and their carers.

Theme 4: Promoting an active, healthy life
Standard 8: The promotion of health and active life in old age. The health and wellbeing of older people is promoted through a coordinated programme of action led by the NHS with support from councils. This standard is linked to the national public health agenda cited above.

Theme 5: Medicines and older people
This is presented as a separate standard to the eight included in the NSF booklet. It recognises the facts that: i) prescribing drugs to the older person needs to take into account how the ageing process affects the body's capacity to handle drugs; ii) multiple diseases and complicated medication regimes may affect patients' capacity and compliance; iii) many adverse reactions are preventable. It recommends

---

BOX 1.1: NSFOP themes and standards—continued

regular review of medicines for all people over age 75 (to ensure that the medicines are producing the desired effect and to detect adverse events), a 'one stop dispensing for discharges' and a scheme by which older people get more help from pharmacists in using their medicines. Specific aspects of medicine use will be discussed in more detail in each chapter of this book.

The National Service Framework for Older People creates opportunities for enhancing the quality of primary care for older people, and general practitioners and primary care nurses with a specialist interest in ageing and health may catalyse change at local level. However, there is a problem of collaboration across professional and agency boundaries, and long-term management of complex problems in older people will inevitably rely on good working relationships between disciplines and organisations. There are many challenges in implementing a public service policy that advocates collaboration between sectors to address both broad quality of life issues as well as health maintenance for older people. The complexities of health and social care partnership working at an organisational level are well documented (Balloch & Taylor 2001), as are those at the service delivery level (Manthorpe & Iliffe 2003), constituting a 'pessimistic tradition' in interprofessional working (Hudson 2002). Trust between disciplines is crucial to collaborative working but may be inhibited if the quality of care varies in one discipline; poor quality general practice makes specialists despair, whilst inconsistent hospital care or hasty discharges with poor discharge planning make general practitioners cynical about their specialist colleagues.

There is a risk that the well-intentioned plans of the National Service Framework for Older People could remain aspirations, for lack of careful thought about how to change services in a policy environment that tries to innovate at ever-greater speed.

How can this be prevented? Expanding on arguments summarised elsewhere (Iliffe & Drennan in press), we suggest that clinicians can reduce the risks of failure by doing what they do best, solving clinical problems. Complex problems usually require complex solutions, which are achieved by sharing knowledge and skills. The great advantage of the National Service Framework is that it sets out not only objectives but also a research and development agenda, since there is much still unknown about how to enhance the quality of care for an ageing population. Specialist and generalist disciplines can rebalance their division of labour, if transfer of skills into primary care can occur and hospital services become more effective in their management of late-life disorders. The lessons from the poor implementation of previous policies (like the '75 and over' checks in general practice) suggest that a cautious and selective approach to chronic disease management, building on existing skills whilst enhancing organisational capability, is the best way to steer between a flurry of policy imperatives and a relatively small, if steadily growing, evidence base. This is what this book attempts to do, by synthesizing the perspectives and approaches of general practitioners and geriatricians to common problems amongst older people.

Chronic disease management

The management of long-term conditions/chronic diseases is the main challenge for primary care worldwide (Bodenheimer et al 2002a). Individuals with long-term conditions consume a large proportion of health and social care resources, including 60%

of hospital bed days in British hospitals (DoH 2004), and 78% of all health care spending in the USA. In North America, comprehensive geriatric assessment with subsequent systematic management reduces hospital admission rates (Stuck et al 2002), and models of chronic disease management have evolved (Bodenheimer et al 2002b) to exploit this impact and contain care costs for an ageing population.

The National Health Service is being encouraged to embark on a chronic disease management (CDM) programme built around fostering self-management, enhancing disease management in primary care, and introducing case management for individuals with complex problems who make high use of hospital services. The Royal Colleges of Physicians, The Royal College of General Practitioners and the NHS Alliance have endorsed this pro-gramme and have made proposals for joint clinical directorates and clinical governance, across the specialist–generalist divide (Royal College of Physicians 2004).

BOX 1.2: Four common chronic clinical problems encountered in the elderly

Arthritis. Arthritis (of several kinds) is the main cause of physical disability in Britain, affecting up to 10 million people, and 70% of those aged 70 years or more. Joint diseases cost the NHS somewhere between £240 and £600 million a year, and care home costs for those with severe disability amount to £130 million.

Diabetes. There are 1.3 million people with diabetes in England alone, and the disease is a major risk factor in heart disease and stroke, as well as a significant cause of renal failure, blindness and peripheral arterial disease severe enough to end in limb amputation.

BOX 1.2: Four common chronic clinical problems encountered in the elderly—continued

Respiratory diseases. Lung diseases other than asthma cause 25% of hospital admissions and 20% of deaths, and three-quarters of the total disease burden are experienced by people aged 65 and over.

Stroke. Stroke is the commonest cause of severe disability and death in the UK, with 110 000 new cases each year in England alone.

The rationale for taking a systematic approach to chronic disease in an ageing population becomes clear when four common clinical problems are considered, as shown in Box 1.2.

The chronic disease management programme has five components, and is based on two assumptions. The two assumptions are that good chronic disease management can improve the quality of life for older people, and that it can also reduce inequalities in health for whole populations. The components are:

1. Undertaking health promotion with older people, to reduce risks of disease and disability.

2. Fostering 'self-management', to give individuals with long-term conditions the knowledge and skills they need to stabilise their health.

3. Systematising disease management for patients with relatively uncomplicated long-term conditions like diabetes or COPD.

4. Introducing case management—the coordination of care across disciplines and agencies—for patients with multiple or complex disabilities.

5. Enhancing knowledge management to identify at-risk groups in the population, carry out needs assessments, understand resource and activity levels and identify trends in health status and service utilisation.

This book focuses on disease management and some aspects of case management of complex problems, but you will also find in it examples of opportunities for health promotion and situations where strengthened self-management would make a positive difference to the experience of ill-health and disability.

In the UK, nurses are seen as the professional discipline with the abilities to carry out and coordinate chronic disease management, and this is seen by the Department of Health as one of the three core roles of primary care nurses. Their contribution is to identify need, achieve continuity of care, promote coherence of services and review the quality of care. This is an important development in the NHS, but one which needs to be explored carefully, for in our view the first question is 'what needs to be done', rather than 'who should do it'. This, we feel, is in keeping with the person-centred approach of the NSFOP, and allows clinicians to begin the process of re-engineering services from the relatively secure base of evidence and practice. There is a risk, we believe, in the premature transfer of tasks to over-worked and under-prepared primary care nurses, who will have little choice but to repeat the error of the '75 and over' checks and adopt an over-simplified check-list approach to complex problems. What we say in this book is couched in medical terminology, but we believe that the key principles of clinical problem solving are shared with, or transferable to, primary care nursing.

We acknowledge that chronic disease management remains problematic as a model of care, with evidence of limited effectiveness, reliance on traditional forms of patient education, poor linkages to primary care and reliance on referrals rather than population-based approaches (Wagner et al 2002). There is also some discussion about whether CDM is wanted by patients, particularly older people who may feel that their independence and autonomy is threatened by an intrusive care system. Finally, there is a question of how to identify those who are likely to need high levels of care, for there is no linear and unambiguous link between the presence of a condition that can be labelled chronic and the need for health or social care (De Lepeleire & Heyrman 2003). These are the issues that we want to address by starting with common clinical problems and exploring ways of solving them by sharing the perspectives and expertise of general practitioners and hospital specialists. We hope that you are as excited by the prospect of doing so as we are, and that this book will assist you in your work.

References

Arber S. Is living longer a cause for celebration? Health Service Journal 1996; 106(5512):28–31.

Balloch S, Taylor M. Partnership working: policy and practice. Bristol: The Policy Press; 2001.

Bodenheimer T, Wagner E, Grumbach K. Improving primary care for patients with chronic illness. JAMA 2002a; 288(14):1775–9.

Bodenheimer T, Wagner E, Grumbach K. Improving primary care for patients with chronic illness: the chronic care model, part 2. JAMA 2002b; 288(15):1909–14.

De Lepeleire J, Heyrman J. Is everyone with a chronic disease also chronically ill? Arch Public Health 2003; 61:161–76.

Department of Health. National Service Framework for Older People. London: HMSO; 2001.

Department of Health. Improving chronic disease management. London: HMSO; 2004.

Fries JF. Ageing, natural death and the compression of morbidity. New Engl J Med 1980; 303(3):130–5.

Hudson B. Interprofessionality in health and social care: the Achilles' heel of partnership. J Interprof Care 2002; 16(1):7–17.

Iliffe S, Drennan V. Assessment of older people in the community: from '75 & over checks' to National Service Frameworks Reviews in Clinical Gerontology 2005 (forthcoming).

Iliffe S, Patterson L, Gould M. Health care for older people. London: BMJ Books; 1998 (pp. 1–5).

Joint working party of RCP(London), RCGP, NHS Alliance. Clinicians, services and commissioning in chronic disease management in the NHS; the need for co-ordinated management programmes. London: Royal College of Physicians; 2004.

Manthorpe J, Iliffe S. Professional predictions: June Huntington's perspectives on joint working, 20 years on. J Interprof Care 2003; 17(1):85–94.

Manton KG, Stalland E, Corder L. Changes in morbidity and chronic disability in the US elderly population: evidence from the 1982, 1984 and 1989 National Long-term Care Survey. J Gerontol B Psychol Sci Soc Sci. 1995; 50(4):S194–204.

Robine JM, Ritchie K. Healthy life expectancy: an evaluation of global indicators of change in population health. BMJ 1991; 302:457–60.

Stuck AE, Egger M, Hammer A, Minder CE, Beck JC. Home visits to prevent nursing home admission and functional decline in the elderly: Systematic review and meta-regression analysis. JAMA 2002; 287(8):1022–8.

Tallis R. Rehabilitation of the elderly in the 21st century. J R Coll Physicians Lond 1992; 26(4):413–22.

Wagner E, Davis C, Schaefer J, Von Korff M, Austin B. A survey of leading chronic disease management programs: are they consistent with the literature? J Nursing Care Qual 2002; 16(2):67–80.

Warnes AM. Elderly people in Great Britain: variable projections and characteristics. Care of the elderly 1989; 1(1):7–10.

Further reading

Grimley Evans J, Goldacre M, Hodleinson H, et al. Health and function in the third age (Carnegie report). London: Nuffield Provincial Hospitals Trust; 1993.

Victor C. Health & health care in later life. Milton Keynes: Open University Press; 1991.

CHAPTER 2

The older patient
with confusion

Mr. C, aged 76, has recently arrived in London from Newcastle upon Tyne to visit his daughter in London. After a few days he becomes confused, acting inappropriately, asking for his deceased wife and not recognising his grandson. His daughter, who has only seen him occasionally over the last 18 months, asks for an urgent appointment with her own general practitioner.

Mr. C's daughter accompanies her father to the GP's surgery to provide background information. She informs the doctor that Mr. C left school at age 16 and joined a major store as a salesman and later became the manager of the local branch. He has smoked since the age of 20 and drinks two units of alcohol per day. He retired at the age of 65 and enjoyed travelling until her mother died three years ago. Although she has seen him every three months or so, she has not noticed anything wrong apart from being 'normal for his age', and nothing unusual had occurred over this period.

The GP finds Mr. C to be fully orientated but a little agitated. Mr. C is able to tell the doctor about his home in Newcastle upon Tyne and his date of birth, but not the present date or month. On physical examination, Mr. C appears well with normal temperature, pulse, blood pressure and no abnormal findings. On testing his urine, the GP notices the presence of blood (++), protein (++) and leucocytes. He sends the sample for culture to the local hospital laboratory and gives Mr. C a prescription for trimethoprim, 200 mg twice a day. That afternoon the GP telephones Mr. C's usual GP in Newcastle upon Tyne to get more details about his previous health. He learns that Mr. C has been a generally healthy man who consults only occasionally, usually with a chest infection in the winter. Next day the GP receives a frantic telephone call from Mr. C's daughter informing him that her father was up all night wandering and at times appeared to hallucinate, seeing flying insects. In view of this deterioration, the GP telephones the registrar on call for medicine of the elderly to discuss the case. The registrar agrees to see the patient for further assessment. In his letter the GP writes:

'Thank you for seeing Mr. C. I feel he has an acute confusional state most likely due to urinary tract infection. In spite of starting oral antibiotics, he is deteriorating and I would appreciate your assessment in order to exclude other pathology to account for his confusion. He is a smoker and I wonder if he could have a chest infection which has not as yet produced clinical signs, or even a bronchogenic carcinoma.'

When she sees Mr. C, the duty medical registrar notes him to be frightened, fidgety and disorientated in time. Physical examination again reveals no abnormalities. In view of the sudden deterioration, the registrar arranges to admit Mr. C for further investigations while continuing with the trimethoprim for a presumed urinary tract infection.

Five days after admission, Mr. C continues to show intermittent confusion. His daughter is concerned by this and asks the GP if he would be willing to contact the hospital and find out what they are doing about his confusion. Dr. GP calls the secretary of the consultant in charge of Mr. C and asks if he could call him back to discuss the case.

The consultant calls back at the end of his morning clinic. He explains that although one would expect the confusion of delirium to resolve with the treatment of a physical illness, the resolution is not always within days. In some it may take longer, and in a minority there may not be improvement in symptoms. In addition, there is always a possibility that he has another pathology or underlying dementia, which is itself a risk factor for developing delirium. It is agreed that since the only abnormality identified so far is a significant growth of *E. coli* in the urine, no additional action is necessary at this stage apart from to continue nursing care while completing the course of antibiotics and providing some mild sedation when required.

Progress

Re-examination on the seventh day reveals brisk reflexes in the left leg with an extensor plantar reflex. In view of this, a CT brain scan is ordered. This reveals no obvious focal abnormality suggestive of a recent cerebrovascular accident but shows changes of small vessel disease and prominence of ventricles and sulci suggestive of cerebral atrophy.

While being investigated, Mr. C's confusion improves and he becomes independent in all activities of daily living. However, he still has difficulty with short-term memory and cannot remember the date. On Mini Mental State Examination (MMSE) he scores 22/30. Further assessment by a clinical psychologist reveals impaired performance in many areas of cognition, and his scores on recognition memory test and on the block design test are below average.

Based on these findings it is concluded that Mr. C had early dementia, probably of the mixed type (Alzheimer's and vascular). Mr. C and his daughter are seen together to discuss the results and are given an information sheet on dementia produced by the Alzheimer's Disease Society. He is started on aspirin 75 mg a day and a referral made to the community mental health nursing team to monitor him, as he has decided to stay with his daughter for at least a couple of months.

LEARNING POINTS FROM CASE HISTORY

○ **Mild dementia may not be obvious to a relative in the early stages and health professionals may not be aware of it unless the person comes to them with a complaint of poor short term memory.**

○ **Dementia is a risk factor for delirium.**

○ **Although delirium usually improves with treatment of underlying physical illness, some features may persist and turn out to be irreversible.**

Tutorial—delirium

Introduction

Delirium is a very common condition, affecting up to 30% of patients presenting to medical services for the elderly. It is associated with high mortality and morbidity in terms of complications, such as falls, pressure sores and continence problems. An episode of delirium may often be the event triggering subsequent institutionalisation of elderly people. It is often not recognised by doctors both in primary care and secondary care settings.

Definition

The main features of delirium according to the Confusional Assessment Method (CAM) include:

1. acute onset of confusion with fluctuating course
2. disorganised thinking—patient may be incoherent or the conversation irrelevant
3. disturbance of consciousness
4. inattention.

To make a diagnosis of delirium the presence of features 1 and 2, and either 3 or 4 are required. It must also be remembered that one in four patients with delirium may not be hyperactive but instead be hypoactive.

Causes can best be remembered using the mnemonic developed by Dr. John E Morley of St. Louis University (Box 2.1).

BOX 2.1: Causes of delirium mnemonic

Drugs—toxicity or side-effects of common drugs such as antidepressants, sedatives etc.
Electrolyte/endocrine problems
Lack of drugs (withdrawal) or low PO_2 states (MI, PE, anaemia, stroke)
Infection, e.g. pneumonia, urinary tract infection
Retention of urine or faeces (impaction)
Intracranial—CVA, TIAs, epilepsy
Under-nutrition/dehydration, urinary retention
Myocardial—ischaemia/infarct, arrhythmias
Subdural haematoma

Patients at risk include those with:

○ pre-existing dementia
○ severe illness
○ physical frailty
○ visual impairment
○ multiple drug therapy (>3 prescribed drugs)
○ excessive alcohol intake.

Delirium is a condition that requires detailed history and thorough physical examination. Investigations will need to be targeted on findings on history and examination. In most cases the following baseline investigation will be relevant:

○ full blood count
○ ESR
○ urea and electrolytes

○ liver function tests

○ calcium and phosphate

○ random glucose

○ thyroid function tests

○ MSU

○ blood culture

○ ECG

○ chest X-ray.

Further investigations (such as CT scan, EEG, etc.) will be determined by findings on history and examination.

If the cause of delirium can be identified with reasonable confidence on clinical grounds and facilities are adequate for care at home (or in a home), it may be appropriate for most of these investigations to be arranged in primary care. Some sedation may be required and the drugs sometimes used would include lorazepam, haloperidol, risperidone or sulpride in low doses. However, in many cases hospital management is required in order to identify, treat and provide 24-hour support for the patient.

Hallucinations may occur in delirium but may suggest other important diagnoses. Common causes of hallucinations in the elderly are listed in Box 2.2. If on assessment the cause is not clear, the patient should be referred for a specialist assessment to a psychiatrist in mental health care of the elderly.

BOX 2.2: Causes of hallucinations in the elderly

- Physiological—occurring on falling asleep (hypnogogic) and on waking (hypnopompic)
- Depression—commonly auditory hallucinations
- Delirium
- Dementia
- Drugs, particularly L-dopa, opiates, antidepressants, steroids
- Bereavement—usually of a dead partner
- Schizophrenia—usually in association with paranoid delusions
- Mania
- Charles Bonnet syndrome (hallucinations that occur in presence of eye pathologies); usually the person is not concerned by the occurrence of hallucinations

Supportive measures in hospital for the patient with delirium

- Nurse in a single room wherever possible.
- Provide frequent reassurance for patient and family.
- If the patient is agitated, try to arrange for a family member or a member of staff to sit with them around the clock.
- Maintain fluid intake and nutrition.
- Minimise sensory deprivation by providing glasses and hearing aids.
- Consider psychotropic drugs (e.g. lorazepam) for patients who are experiencing considerable distress and are at risk to themselves or others around them.

KEY LEARNING POINTS—DELIRIUM

○ Delirium is common in the elderly.

○ It is associated with increased morbidity (prolonged hospital stay, increased risk of pressure sores, falls, infections and increased risk of institutionalisation) and mortality.

○ As an acute condition it is usually best managed in hospital.

Tutorial—dementia

Size of problem

Dementia is one of the common problems of old age with a reported prevalence of 5% over the age of 65. In the UK it is estimated that there are over 700,000 people affected by dementia and this figure is likely to rise to 1.2 million by 2040. The impact of dementia is not only on the sufferer but also on the family/carers and on health, social and voluntary services. In the UK dementia has been estimated to cost the community £2.4 billion per year.

Types of dementia

As a clinical syndrome dementia can be caused by a number of specific disease entities. The five most common are listed in Box 2.3.

BOX 2.3: The five common types of dementia

- Alzheimer's disease (AD)
- Vascular dementia (VD)
- Mixed type dementia (AD and VD)
- Lewy body dementia
- Frontal/frontotemporal dementia

Table 2.1: General features suggestive of dementia	
Cognitive	• Sustained decline in memory • Difficulty in handling complex tasks • Difficulty in reasoning • Language problems • Impairment in spatial and visuo-perceptual ability
Non-cognitive	• Changes in behaviour • Changes in emotional control • Changes in social functioning

Clinical features

Dementia usually starts with a gradual memory impairment, predominantly for recent events. The individual, their family and sometime their doctor may put this down at first to 'normal ageing'. Formal diagnosis is often not made until the condition is advanced, with one or more of the feature/symptoms listed in Table 2.1. In addition to these general features, the presence of particular features will support the diagnosis of a specific type of dementia. These are listed in Table 2.2.

Assessment by the GP at home

Any person presenting with memory difficulties requires not only assessment of memory and cognition but physical examination and baseline investigations to exclude reversible causes (Box 2.4) and non-dementing causes of memory difficulties and confusion, such as depression and also delirium, where the onset is usually acute (see above).

Table 2.2: Features suggestive of specific types of dementia	
Vascular dementia	• Abrupt onset • Stepwise progression of disease process • Focal neurological symptoms and signs • Presence of arteriosclerosis • Nocturnal confusion • Associated atherosclerosis and hypertension
Lewy body dementia	• Fluctuating impairment of cognition with variations in alertness and attention • Visual hallucinations • Parkinsonism • Increased sensitivity to neuroleptics • Repeated falls • Systemised delusions • Disturbance of consciousness
Frontotemporal dementia	• Syndrome of frontotemporal lobal degeneration • Onset in the mid to late fifties but can be between 45 and 70 • Insidious onset • Loss of personal awareness with neglect in personal hygiene, dishevelled appearance, disinhibition (making lewd or sexual remarks), lack of empathy, impulsivity, executive dysfunction, loss of insight, bizarre disconnected affect
Progressive non-fluent aphasia	• Syndrome of frontotemporal lobal degeneration • Degeneration of frontal cortex leading to progressive worsening of nonfluent spontaneous speech with agrammatism, phonemic paraphasia, and anomia • Patients may preserve social skills in early stages

---

BOX 2.4: Tests recommended for detecting reversible causes
of dementia

- Full blood count
- Thyroid function (hypothyroidism, thyrotoxicosis)
- Bone biochemistry (hypercalcaemia)
- Vitamin B_{12} deficiency
- Folate deficiency
- Liver function tests (alcohol)
- Serology for syphilis
- CT scan of brain (normal pressure hydrocephalus /tumour)

Depression is common in people with dementia, particularly those with vascular dementia. It is estimated that 12% of patients with dementia suffer from depression. Severe depression may produce features suggestive of dementia ('pseudo-dementia'), which improve with treatment with antidepressants. It is worth remembering that often depression may not be obvious because it presents with atypical features in people with dementia; symptoms such as aggressive behaviour, refusal of food or medication, wandering, apathy or insomnia may herald the onset of depression. Treatment of depression will often improve symptoms. See Chapter 5 for a full discussion of depression in older people.

The brief assessments of cognition that are easy to administer in the community include the Abbreviated Mental Test Score, Mini-mental State Examination of Folstein (see below), Clock Drawing test and Middlesex Elderly Assessment of Mental State.

M M S E

MMSE is a brief measure of cognitive function, and areas assessed by the text include orientation to time and place (10 points), registration of three words (3 points), attention and calculation (5 points), word recall (3 points), language (8 points), and visual construction (1 point). The scores range from 0 to 30, and for people with more than eight years of education, a score of 23 or less is usually indicative of cognitive impairment.

When to refer to hospital

After baseline investigations have excluded reversible causes, the person with abnormal results on cognition testing and those with normal results on screening but who continue to complain of memory difficulties, should be referred for specialist multi-professional assessment, which may include examination by a physician or a psychiatrist with interest in mental health care of older people, and a psychologist.

The role of the specialist team is:

o To quantify the memory and cognitive difficulties in those who have abnormal results on screening and to detect early subtle change of cognition in those with normal screening tests.

o To consider further investigations using neuro-imaging such as CT or MRI. These scans, although not diagnostic, will help support the diagnosis of dementia and more importantly exclude other causes, such as tumour or normal pressure hydrocephalus.

o To identify the type of dementia, since management of the dementia syndrome and its features depend upon making an accurate diagnosis.

○ To advise the patient how best to cope with the memory difficulties.

○ To offer treatment based on available evidence.

○ To help support the person and his/her family at home, jointly with the general practitioner.

Management at home

Patients with dementia will require support and services at all stages of the disease process. The exact need will be determined by the circumstances of the individual and family, and the range of support will be dependent upon locally available services.

During the early stages, advice, education and counselling are important, and in this respect a person should be advised to contact an organisation such as the Alzheimer's Disease Society.

Social support may also be needed by some individuals during the early stages, but this is usually required more as the disease progresses and the patient's needs change. The range of support available in most districts includes CPN monitoring, carer/patient counselling, respite care, day hospital, psychiatric care support programmes, social services (such as meals on wheels) and home care for basic activities such as washing, bathing, dressing, cleaning and shopping.

At some stage, support in the community may become inadequate for a person with advanced dementing illness. When this happens, placement in a residential home or nursing home with beds for elderly mentally infirm may become inevitable, and in some individuals this can be a positive step not only for the patient but the carers.

Medical management by the GP will require coordination of all services/supports mentioned above, especially in dealing with physical illnesses that may arise since these are likely to lead to development of delirium on top of dementia and, therefore, worsening of the features of dementia.

Behavioural and psychiatric symptoms can be treated at home using anti-psychotic agents, such as sulpiride, risperidone, trazodone or even rivastigmine, but once simple antipsychotic agents fail to work, input from a specialist should be sought. Certainly drug treatment for patients with Lewy body dementia should be monitored by a specialist, as these patients are very prone to developing side-effects.

In addition to treating the behavioural symptoms, it is important to treat vascular risk factors (e.g. hypertension), as there is some evidence that these factors play a causal role in cognitive decline in all types of dementia.

Non-medical management

Non-medical approaches, such as cognitive therapy, emotion-based approaches or behavioural therapy, can also help patients with dementia but require the input of an experienced psychologist.

Management at hospital

Management by specialists is required for initiation and monitoring of pharmacological treatment, particularly for patients with dementia of Alzheimer's type. There are currently four available drugs (Table 2.3), three of which are useful (NICE 2001) in patients with mild to moderate degree of dementia (MMSE > 12), while the fourth (memantine) is said to be

Table 2.3: Drugs available for Alzheimer's type of dementia

Drug	Dose	Side-effects
Donepezil—a selective reversible inhibitor of AchE[2]	5–10 mg od	Nausea, vomiting, diarrhoea, headache, dizziness, fatigue, psychiatric disturbances, insomnia, urinary incontinence, muscle cramps, rash, pruritus and less frequently bradycardias, convulsions, gastric/duodenal ulcers and gastrointestinal haemorrhage
Rivastigmine—pseudo-irreversible inhibitor of AchE	3–6 mg bd	As above, although gastric/duodenal ulcers occur rarely + tremor, abdominal pain, pancreatitis, asthenia, agitation, sweating, insomnia, hallucinations, hypertension, cardiac arrhythmias, pancreatitis (rare)
Galantamine—AchE inhibitor and potentiator of nicotinic responses induced by Ach	8–12 mg bd	As for donepezil + abdominal pain, dizziness, rhinitis, syncope, bladder outflow obstruction
Memantine—N-methyl-D-aspartate (NMDA) receptor antagonist	10 mg bd	Dizziness, vertigo, fatigue, confusion, hallucinations, headache, diarrhoea and gastric pain and less commonly vomiting, anxiety, cystitis, increased libido and hypertonia

indicated for use in those with moderately severe to severe Alzheimer's disease. It is important to explain to patients and families that these drugs do not cure dementia. They may lead to improvement in cognitive and non-cognitive symptoms and signs, but more likely just to a slowing down of the dementia process, particularly delaying the onset of advanced symptoms that may lead to institutionalisation.

Conditions which are relative contraindications to such therapy include:

o gastrointestinal diseases causing vomiting or diarrhoea

o bradycardia

o chronic airflow limitation

o benign prostatic hypertrophy.

In the later stages of dementia (i.e. in patients with moderately severe or severe Alzheimer's disease), memantine, an NMDA (N-methyl-D-aspartate) receptor antagonist, has been shown to improve activities of daily living, thus helping the individuals to avoid/delay entry to nursing home care. However, data on memantine is lacking, and at best the drug seems only to produce a small reduction in the rate of deterioration in global, functional and cognitive scales. The commonly reported side-effects of memantine include hallucinations, confusion, dizziness, tiredness and headache.

In addition to acetyl cholinesterase inhibitors, patients with Alzheimer's diseases as well those with vascular dementia may benefit from vitamin C and vitamin E, free radical scavengers or gingko biloba preparation.

In the later stages of dementia hospital input may be required to stabilise therapy for symptom control, such as intractable behavioural problems, or where there are complex family relationship difficulties or if psychotic or depressive episodes do not respond to treatment or for assessment of a person's needs in the late stages of disease. Of course management at this stage will require good communication between the family and professionals working in hospital and community.

ROLE OF OESTROGENS AND ANTI-INFLAMMATORY DRUGS IN ALZHEIMER'S DISEASE

While there is epidemiological evidence supporting the protective effects of oestrogens and anti-inflammatory agents, they are not recommended as part of routine management at the present time.

Difficult decisions faced by general practitioners

1. INFORMING THE PATIENT AND FAMILY OF THE DIAGNOSIS

In medicine, ethical dilemmas most often arise from conflict between moral imperatives, such as telling the truth, and doing no harm. However, issues of consent to investigations and treatment require disclosure of diagnosis. This applies to dementia, unless the disease process has progressed to the stage at which the patient is incapable of understanding what is being discussed.

Sometimes relatives may know or suspect the diagnosis and ask the doctor not to disclose it. However, it is important to explain to the family that a competent adult has the moral and legal right to know the diagnosis and be involved in any decisions about investigation, treatment and future care.

In medico-legal terms, a person is judged competent if they are over age 16 and are able to:

o understand and retain the information given to them
o believe the information
o weigh up the risks and benefits to arrive at a decision.

2. MENTAL CAPACITY

As the disease process progresses, individuals become increasingly less able to handle their personal and financial affairs. Therefore, it is important to advise patients in the early stages of dementia, when they still have the capacity to understand and make decisions, to seriously consider making an Enduring Power of Attorney (EPA). An EPA is a legal document that enables an individual (the donor) to appoint one or more persons (attorney) to manage his or her financial affairs and property, either now or in the future. When the individual loses the capacity to manage affairs, the Enduring Power of Attorney loses its validity but allows the attorney to register it with a Court of Protection.

The Mental Capacity Act, which has just received the Royal Assent, will create a new power of attorney ('the lasting power of attorney') that will allow a person to appoint an attorney to make decision on welfare, including health and financial affairs. This new provision will replace the EPA. The Act will also allow the court to appoint deputies to make decisions on behalf of a person about matters in relation to which that person lacks capacity, and will create independent 'mental capacity advocates' to support and represent people lacking capacity who have no one else to speak for them when decisions need to be taken about serious medical treatment and long-term residential care.

Sometimes a doctor is asked to comment on an individual's capacity for making a will. In assessing 'testamentary capacity', the doctor must ensure that the person:

○ knows the nature of the action of making a will

○ has a reasonable grasp of his/her assets

○ knows the person(s) to whom he/she is leaving his/her assets

○ is free of delusions that might affect judgement.

3. DEMENTIA AND NEGLECT

Personal neglect is common in the stages of disease, particularly in those who are living alone. This may result from the presence of an acute illness or may result from the progression of the disease itself. Section 47 of the National Assistance Act 1948 can be used to admit a person to hospital on a temporary basis when he/she is not able to look after him/herself (but this does not allow treatment to be given). A person can also be moved for a longer period of time into a safer environment using 'guardianship' under the Mental Health Act 1983. The 'guardian' appointed by a local authority has the power to require the individual to live at a particular safe place, to gain access for doctors, social workers for treatment and to require the patient to attend at set times for medical treatment.

4. DEMENTIA AND DRIVING

Dementia can affect driving through changes in judgement, visuo-spatial difficulties and inattentiveness, and there is evidence that a diagnosis of dementia is associated with increased risk of accidents. In the early stages, the person may not have any difficulty with driving, but as the disease progresses and the dementia becomes moderate, the patient should be advised to stop driving until there can be a full assessment by a psychologist or Driving Licensing Authorities. If a person refuses to accept advice, the doctor may report this to DVLA under the 1988 Road Traffic Act.

5. ISSUES SURROUNDING GENETIC TESTING

Some relatives may ask or demand presymptomatic testing, particularly if there is familial Alzheimer's disease. The advice at the present time is that, as there are no preventive or protective treatments currently available, genetic testing is not indicated, particularly as it can have grave psychological implications for the individual and family members.

6. ADVICE TO CARERS OF A PERSON WITH DEMENTIA

○ Contact a local and or national Alzheimer's disease society.

○ Simplify the environment (house or flat) the patient is living in.

○ Provide a bracelet with name, address and carer's telephone number in case the patient wanders and gets lost.

○ Ensure the patient follows advice on driving.

○ Protect the individual's finances (see above for Lasting Power of Attorney and Court of Protection).

○ Simplify daily routine.

○ Reduce the likelihood of confusion and restlessness by using good lighting.

○ Avoid startling a patient who has a tendency to develop behavioural symptoms.

○ Ensure compliance with medication.

○ Keep the individual's mind active by encouraging regular interests.

KEY LEARNING POINTS—DEMENTIA

- Patients complaining of memory problems, particularly for recent events, should be assessed using the Mini-Mental State Examination (MMSE) or Abbreviated Mental Test (AMT) and screened for treatable causes of dementia-like syndrome.

- Those with normal MMSE/AMT results and normal screening for treatable conditions should be reassessed six months later, and if complaint of memory difficulty persists should be referred to hospital for further assessment.

- Those with abnormal MMSE scores should be referred to a physician with an interest in dementia, or a psychiatrist specialising in the mental health care of older people.

- During early stages, education and counselling are important, as is initiation of treatment with anticholinesterase inhibitors in case of Alzheimer's disease, or vitamin C or E as anti-oxidants and gingko preparations for vascular dementia.

- Treatment with anticholinesterase inhibitors will require monitoring by specialists.

- Psychological treatment may be useful but will require referral to an experienced psychologist.

- In late stages, behavioural problems may require use of antipsychotic agents. If first-line drugs, such as risperidone or sulpiride, fail to control symptoms then help from a specialist should be sought.

- With the progression of the disease, medico-legal issues (with assessment of mental capacity, neglect and driving) may become important.

- The family of any patient with dementia will need ongoing support and advice with respect to both medical management and social care.

Further reading

National Institute for Clinical Excellence. Technology Appraisal Guidance no. 19. Guidance on the use of donepezil, rivastigmine and gallantamine for the treatment of Alzheimer's disease. London: National Institute for Clinical Excellence; 2001. **www.nice.org.uk.**

Gleason OC. Delirium. Am Fam Physician 2003; 67: 1027–1034.

Grossberg GT, Desai AK. Management of Alzheimer's disease. J Gerontol 2003; 58A:331–353.

CHAPTER 3

The older patient with falls

CASE HISTORY

Mrs. F is 80 years old. One morning her neighbour calls the GP surgery to say she is worried about her. Mrs. F had fallen over the day before and hurt her back. Although Mrs. F does not seem badly hurt, the neighbour is worried because she has fallen several times recently and has now become afraid of going out. The GP agrees that Mrs. F will need medical assessment and tells the neighbour that he will arrange to see her that day. He telephones Mrs. F who says she has only tripped and fallen accidentally once or twice. However, she agrees to see him as she hasn't been feeling well. As Mrs. F cannot get to the surgery, the GP agrees that he will visit her that afternoon.

The GP has known this patient over the years to be relatively uncomplaining, but he notes that during recent months she has been seen quite often with a variety of minor complaints, and that she is now on four different medications and apparently having increasing difficulty looking after herself.

When the GP visits, he notices that Mrs. F takes some time getting to the door to let him in. He is certain she has lost weight. He goes through her problems with her, and she tells him that she is especially troubled by giddiness first thing in the morning when she gets out of bed. She also describes difficulty getting in and out of her bath. Having fallen over in the street on two occasions, she now feels too anxious to go out, and staying in on her own is making her feel quite depressed. He notes her medication to be amitriptyline 50 mg, co-amilozide × 1, aspirin 75 mg, and thyroxine 0.1 mg daily.

While examining Mrs. F, the GP notices that she is very thin and having some difficulty getting out of her chair, needing to hold on to the arms. Her blood pressure is 150/70, dropping to 130/80 on standing. Her pulse rate is 80 beats per minute. Her heart sounds are normal and her chest is clear, but she does have some ankle swelling. She also has some osteoarthritis of her right hip.

The GP decides first of all that she needs some blood tests, an ECG and probably a chest X-ray. Her medication also needs rationalisation, as it is probably causing postural hypotension. He is sure she would also benefit from assessment by a physiotherapist and dietician. An eye test would also be helpful, as poor vision may be contributing to her tripping and falling.

He discusses with her the best way to arrange these things. They agree that it would be very difficult for her to go separately for all the tests and assessments, and that she would prefer to be referred to the Falls Clinic at the local day hospital for older people.

At the Falls Clinic she is seen by the specialist registrar in elderly medicine who takes a detailed history and examines her thoroughly. The registrar agrees that postural hypotension and visual impairment are likely to be the main causes of her falls, possibly aggravated by gait disturbance due to her osteoarthritis. The registrar arranges the following investigations: FBC, ESR, U&E, glucose, LFT, TFT, B_{12}, chest X-ray, resting and 24-hour ECG. She also organises physiotherapy, dietetics and optometry assessments and refers Mrs. F to the occupational therapist for a home visit.

The registrar is also concerned that Mrs. F is taking a strong loop diuretic, as well as a tricyclic antidepressant. As Mrs. F still seems depressed, the registrar replaces the tricyclic antidepressant with a serotonin reuptake inhibitor (SSRI) and considers stopping the diuretic altogether. However, since there is still some ankle swelling and a risk that she could develop further symptoms, the registrar decides initially to switch from co-amilozide to bumetanide, as this is a longer-acting diuretic less likely to cause postural hypotension.

The occupational therapist goes on a home visit and identifies some environmental hazards. She suggests rearrangement of some rugs and carpets, and arranges for the installation of handrails up the stairs and at the side of Mrs. F's bath and toilet. The physiotherapist arranges for Mrs. F to attend a strength and balance retraining programme and encourages her to join a falls group to continue to build-up her strength. The optometrist identifies cataracts, and Mrs. F is referred to ophthalmology to consider removal.

Three months later Mrs. F is back to her old self. Her postural hypotension has disappeared, her cataracts have been removed and she is managing to do her own shopping and visit friends locally.

LEARNING POINTS FROM CASE HISTORY

- **Any elderly patient with falls requires detailed assessment with particular attention to the history.**
- **Many older people who fall have retrospective amnesia for the event and will rationalise the reason for falling.**
- **Sometimes a third-party history is required to ensure accuracy of the history.**
- **Simple examination and investigation are useful in excluding several treatable causes of falls.**

Tutorial — falls

This tutorial will initially describe the definition and incidence of falls. It will examine the risk factors for and causes of falls. It will go on to describe the assessment and management of fallers in the primary care sector and those who might benefit from a referral to secondary care. Finally, we will consider the benefit of interventions to prevent falls in the elderly.

Definition and incidence of falls

In 1987, the Kellogg's International Working Group on Falls defined a fall as 'unintentionally coming to the ground or some lower level other than as a consequence of sustaining a violent blow, loss of consciousness, sudden onset of paralysis as in stroke or an epileptic seizure'. Since then researchers have used a broader definition to include those that occur as a result of dizziness and syncope. Falls are one of the most common and serious problems which older people face. They are associated with considerable mortality and morbidity, a reduction in functioning/activities in daily living and hence an increased likelihood of premature admission to care home. Of those aged 65 and over, 35–40% fall annually. Fifty per cent of these falls occur in the home and immediate home surroundings. People over age 75 have a much higher rate, and those living in care homes or hospital have three times the rate of falling in comparison with those living in the community. Each year, 135,000 people aged over 75 fall, costing the NHS £1.7 billion per year. The importance of primary, secondary and tertiary prevention of falls has been recognised in the National Service Framework (NSF) for older people (Standard 6). This recommends that a 'falls service' should be available in every primary care trust.

It should provide an integrated service to improve care and prevention of serious injury from falls, as well as long-term rehabilitation.

Risk factors and causes of falls

Older people fall as a consequence of multiple, diverse risk factors and situations, many of which are remediable (Box 3.1). These risk factors are also influenced by age, disease, presence of environmental hazards and a lack of awareness of falling. Risk factors for falling are often not recognised by either professionals or by the sufferers themselves. Factors that increase the likelihood of falling include:

- acute and chronic ill health
- presense of multiple diseases
- poor strength and balance
- impaired cognition
- multiple use of medication
- poor lighting
- environmental hazards such as rugs
- inadequate foot wear
- alcohol intake
- poor vision and hearing.

BOX 3.1: Risk factors for fall

- Muscle weakness
- History of falls
- Gait deficit
- Balance deficit
- Use of assisted device

BOX 3.1: Risk factors for fall—continued

- Visual deficit
- Arthritis
- Impaired activity of daily living
- Depression
- Cognitive impairment
- Age over 80
- Cardiovascular disease

The NICE guidelines for falls (April 2004) and the AGS/BGS guidelines (2001) on falls (Fig. 3.1) recommend routine questioning in older people about falls in the last year. The AGS/BGS guidelines recommend the following approach as part of routine care (not presenting after a fall):

1. All older persons who are under the care of a health professional should be asked at least once a year about falls.
2. All older persons who report a single fall should be observed as they stand up from a chair without using their arms and walk several paces in return (i.e. the get up and go test). Those demonstrating no difficulty or unsteadiness need no further assessment.
3. People who have difficulty or demonstrate unsteadiness performing this test require further assessment.

It is recommended that general practitioners and primary care teams should record the following to identify fallers or those at risk of falling:

- ○ trouble with walking
- ○ feeling off balance

○ weakness and problems with legs

○ use of walking stick, walking aid or walker

○ documentation of visual problems

○ information about the number of medications.

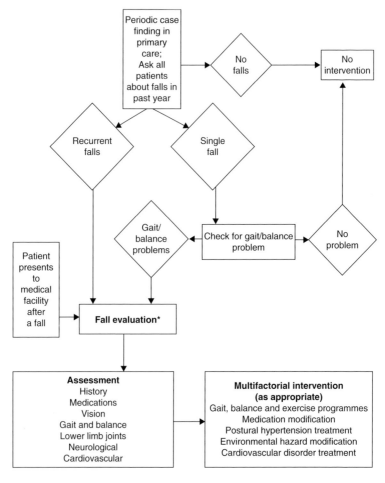

Fig. 3.1: Case finding in primary care. Algorithm summarising the assessment and management of falls.

Older people are more likely to fall if they are frail, find the activities of daily living difficult, have been recently discharged from hospital and are on more than four medications. Older people who fall not only have a greater susceptibility to injury but have a high prevalence of co-morbid disease, for example osteoporosis and age-related physiological decline. Falls in old age are caused by an interaction of intrinsic, extrinsic and environmental factors. The intrinsic factors include sensory deficits, orthostatic hypotension, gait and balance changes, musculoskeletal changes, cognitive impairment, cardiovascular problems and medication. Extrinsic/environmental causes include trips or accidents which may be due to poor lighting, clutter, loose rugs, ill-fitting clothes, wires and wet floors. Table 3.1 provides an example of a classification of falls by cause.

Consequences of falls

Falls are the principal cause of injury leading to hospital admission and death amongst over-65s in the United Kingdom. Two percent of falls are fatal, and six percent result in bone fractures of which 25% are hip fractures. Head injury, lacerations and other soft tissue injuries are also common. Prolonged waits on the floor after falling put elderly patients at risk of hypothermia, pressure sores, dehydration, pulmonary embolism and pneumonia.

In institutional care, 10–25% of older people who fall will develop a fracture or laceration or the need for hospital care. In general, fall-related injuries account for 6% of all medical expenditure for older people aged over 65. Five per cent of older fallers require hospitalisation. Falls are the fifth leading cause of death, and recurrent falls are a common reason for admission to long-term care (one study showed that 40% of nursing home admissions had been precipitated by falls).

Table 3.1: Classification of falls by aetiology

Sensory deficits	Visual impairment Vestibular problems
Nervous system	TIA Stroke Parkinsonism Dementia Ataxia Epilepsy Upper motor neurone lesions Peripheral nerve lesions Cervical spondylosis/myelopathy Neuropathy
Musculoskeletal	Weakness/deconditioning Arthritis Osteoporosis/osteomalacia Myelopathy Previous fracture Foot/shoe problems
Cardiovascular	Postural hypotension Arrhythmia Angina Cardiac failure Anaemia
Intoxications/Medication	Hypotensives Diuretics Antidepressants Hypnotics/anxiolytics More than four of any medications ETOH or drug abuse
Intercurrent acute illness	Especially febrile illness, e.g. UTI, chest infection Hypothermia
Haematological/ biochemical disorders	Anaemia Hypoglycaemia Hypokalaemia Hyponatraemia
Extrinsic causes	Trips and accidents

Assessment of fallers

The clinical assessment of any patient presenting with one or more falls should include attention to the following:

○ history and circumstances of the fall

○ any loss of consciousness

○ any loss of movement or involuntary movement

○ any incontinence

○ all prescribed and over-the-counter medications

○ any recent acute and/or ongoing chronic medical problems

○ any previous problems with gait and balance

○ chest pain

○ palpitations

○ hearing problems

○ eye sight problems

○ memory loss

○ depression

○ habits relating to alcohol or recreational drugs.

Physical examination should focus initially on seeking signs of acute injury due to the fall. After this, look in every system for clues to acute or chronic conditions which may predispose to falling. Observation of gait, balance and vision should be part of this examination. It should also include the 'get up and go' test. This should be supplemented by evaluation of the function and strength of the patient's legs. The cardiovascular system should be examined, including heart rate/rhythm (potential arrhythmias), the lying and standing blood pressure, heart sounds for murmur of aortic stenosis and gallop rhythms, and carotids for bruits. Carotid sinus stimulation should be performed when appropriate. There should be an assessment of lower extremity joint function. A basic examination of the neurological system should include mental status, nystagmus, muscle strength, lower extremity peripheral nerves, proprioception, reflexes, cortical, extrapyramidal and cerebellar function. Extremities examination should include the feet for corns, callus, bunions, long nails, ulcers and ill-fitting shoes.

Laboratory investigations should include FBC, ESR, U&E, glucose, LFT, TFT, B_{12}, chest X-ray and resting ECG. These simple tests will exclude many of the causes of falls listed in Table 3.2. A 24-hour tape is required when there is a possibility of a blackout/syncope secondary to an arrhythmia or heart block. An echocardiogram is useful if aortic stenosis or HOCM (hypertrophic obstructive cardiomyopathy) is suspected.

Management of fallers

Further management of any patient with falls will clearly be guided by the findings from the history, examination and investigation, such that any identified risk factors or causes of falling can be specifically addressed. Much of the management focuses on prevention of further falls (see below). This will always include a careful review of the risks and benefits of any medication which the patient is currently taking. Physiotherapy and occupational therapy can be helpful in identifying and reducing environmental risks for falling. Strength and balance exercises can help individuals learn to get up after a fall. The patient's family and social services can help in terms of support and monitoring, and may be able to provide alarm systems so that the patient can call for help in the event of a fall when alone.

FALLS PREVENTION

The most effective approach in the prevention of falls has been shown to be a multi-factorial falls risk assessment and management programme with multi-disciplinary interventions. The assessment and management programme should include medication review, with modification and rationalisation where required. It should also include regular physical exercise, muscle strengthening and balance retraining, as well as home hazard assessment. In the UK, such an assessment can be undertaken in a 'falls clinic' provided by the local department of elderly medicine.

One of the most successful interventions is the rationalisation of medications. This is made more difficult because older patients tend to have multiple pathology. Changes of medication should be implemented with a proper explanation, and patients should be carefully followed-up.

Cardiac pacing is indicated for carotid sinus syndrome and heart block, whereas the older person who has paroxysmal arrhythmias requires appropriate treatment. Older patients where postural hypotension is diagnosed may require modification and reduction of either cardiac or neuroleptic drugs. Tai chi for balance retraining has been found to be effective in the prevention of falls. Hip protectors are useful in those at risk from hip fractures.

In long-term care settings, staff education, gait retraining, review of medications with particular attention to psychotropic medication can be helpful. Assisted devices (such as bed alarms, canes, Zimmer frames and hip protectors) have been found to be useful.

Calcium and vitamin D can be helpful in those at risk from vitamin deficiency. Obviously, older people are more at risk from osteoporosis, and osteoporosis guidelines should be followed (Box 3.2). Appropriate footwear should always be recommended, and staff in care homes should be encouraged not to use restraint, either medically or physically, because of the severe negative consequences.

BOX 3.2: Secondary prevention of osteoporotic fragility fractures in post-menopausal women: NICE guidelines 2004

- Prevention of fragility fractures in those who have sustained a fracture. Bisphosphonates recommended without need for DEXA scan in those aged over 75.
- Recommended if osteoporosis is demonstrated on a DEXA scan 65–75.
- Raloxifene is recommended second line if bisphosphonates are contraindicated.
- Calcium and vitamin D recommended if low dietary intake or at risk of vitamin D deficiency.

At present, there is insufficient evidence for the benefits of low-intensity exercise, group exercise, and cognitive and behavioural interventions. Older patients should be encouraged to tell their doctors when they fall and the circumstances of the fall. They should be made aware of the benefits from preventing falls, and should be encouraged to be in partnership with the primary care team to prevent further falls.

Many interventions have been developed to prevent falls. Systematic reviews have not reached conclusions on the absolute effectiveness of individual components of these interventions, and the relative effectiveness of different approaches to prevent falls is also unknown. Exercise programmes include both general and specific physical activities. Examples of general activities include walking, cycling and anaerobic movements. Specific activity includes training targeted towards balance, gait and strength.

Environmental modification programmes which include home visits to check for environmental hazards are described above.

KEY LEARNING POINTS—FALLS

○ Ill health or frailty in old age can often present with a fall.

○ General practitioners and specialists when seeing older people should always take a 'falls' history.

○ Risk factors for falls include multiple medications, depression, dementia, poor eyesight, giddiness, unsteadiness and difficulty with walking.

○ Patients presenting with falls should be fully investigated to identify treatable causes of falls.

○ The NICE guidelines for falls are a useful aide to management (see National Institute for Clinical Excellence citation below).

References

American Geriatrics Society, British Geriatrics Society and American Academy of Orthopaedic Surgeons Panel on Falls Prevention. Guidelines for the prevention of falls in older persons. J Am Geriatr Soc 2001; 49(5):664–672.

Kellogg International Work Group on the Prevention of Falls by the Elderly report. The prevention of falls in later life. Dan Med Bull 1987; 34(Suppl 4):1–24.

National Institute for Clinical Excellence. Clinical Guideline 21, Falls: the assessment and prevention of falls in older people. November 2004. **www.nice.org.uk.**

Further reading

Gillespie L. Preventing falls in elderly people. BMJ 2004; 328(7441):653–654.

Tinetti ME. Clinical practice. Preventing falls in elderly persons. N Engl J Med 2003; 348(1):42–49.

CHAPTER 4

The older patient with mobility problems

Mrs. MP is an 80-year-old woman who lives alone. Her daughter, who lives in another town, phones up her mother's GP surgery asking for a visit to her mother as she is worried about her. The GP telephones back to Mrs. MP's daughter to get some more information and ask if she could perhaps come to the surgery. The daughter tells him that Mrs. MP has been deteriorating over the last few months. She had visited her mother that week and was most distressed to see that she is now completely housebound and having great difficulty coping. The GP remembers how uncomplaining Mrs. MP normally was, and he agrees to visit her later that day.

General practitioner visit

On arrival at her home, the GP waits a long time for the door to be answered. When Mrs. MP eventually arrives, he sees that she is moving with difficulty and appears to be in pain. They sit in her living room and she tells him that she has terrible pain in her left knee. On further questioning it seems she has low energy and is breathless on the slightest exertion but not on lying down. She is finding increasing difficulty getting out of bed and on and off her chair. She is not feeling well enough to go out on her own and feels very lonely and fed-up. On examination, the GP finds that she has swelling and a valgus deformity of her left knee, reduced movement around her left hip, swollen ankles, long dirty toe nails and dirty feet. While being examined, she admits that she is no longer able to get into the bath or cut her toenails. Her neighbour is doing the shopping but she can manage to make her own meals.

On examination, she has no signs of anaemia, no goitre, a normal pulse and a slightly raised blood pressure. Her lungs are clear, and abdominal and brief neurological examinations are unremarkable. She is a little deaf but there is no evidence of cognitive impairment. The GP decides that Mrs. MP needs some further investigations in order to make a full assessment. He feels she needs a full blood count and ESR (to rule out polymyalgia rheumatica, in particular), thyroid function tests in case she has become hypothyroid, U&E, ECG, a chest X-ray to further assess possible hypertension or ischaemic heart disease, and an X-ray of her hips and knees to confirm his suspicion of significant osteoarthritis. Given her poor mobility and lack of local family support, the GP and the patient agree that the best plan is a referral to the local day hospital for older people where she can have all the necessary tests and assessments by a specialist, a nurse, a physiotherapist, an occupational therapist and a dietician.

The GP also wonders if Mrs. MP has become depressed as a consequence of her pain and isolation. He discusses this with her, and they agree to talk about the possibility of counselling and/or possible antidepressant medication once they have more information about her physical problems. Meanwhile, he also discusses with Mrs. MP if she would be willing to be referred to social services, who could arrange an assessment with a view to arranging meals on wheels and perhaps a home carer. She can also think about attending a lunch club or bingo once or twice a week for a change of scene and to meet some other people. The GP dictates referral letters to both the day hospital and social services that same day, and they are faxed through the following morning.

Day hospital (assessment by multidisciplinary team)

At the day hospital, Mrs. MP is first seen by the SHO in elderly medicine. A full history is taken and a thorough examination performed.

Mrs. MP admits that she had not wished to worry her GP or her daughter and, therefore, had not mentioned to them additional problems, including low back ache which is limiting her mobility. She also tells the SHO that recently she had called out an emergency doctor who had prescribed her temazepam to help her sleep because she was in so much pain. On examination, in addition to her arthritis, she is found to be quite obese, weighing 70 kg, and she has swelling of the ankles which is thought to be dependent oedema. She also has tenderness over her lumbar spine and reduced straight leg raising on the left. The SHO discusses the case with her consultant. They agree on the necessary investigations and a plan to encourage her, meanwhile, to take paracetamol on a more regular basis (two tablets every six hours) and to gradually withdraw the temazepam, which may be making her drowsy in the daytime and (given her poor mobility) putting her at risk of falls. They decide that a time-limited course of non-steroidal inflammatory drugs is not advisable because she does suffer with occasional heartburn. She is also assessed by the physiotherapist (who recommends retraining with particular emphasis on quadriceps strengthening exercises) and the occupational therapist, who arranges a follow-up visit to her home in order to look at the possibility of providing equipment to make her bed and chair transfers more easier.

Mrs. MP is seen again at the day hospital one week later with the results of her tests. X-rays confirm the diagnosis of severe osteoarthritis in the left hip and the left knee, and degenerative changes of her lumbar spine. Her ESR is normal, but she is biochemically hypothyroid. Other investigations reveal no significant abnormalities. After taking a further blood sample to check her thyroid antibodies, she is commenced on thyroxine and arrangements are made for follow-up to check her response to treatment. She is seen by the dietician, who provides her with advice on healthy eating, and by the podiatrist, who cuts her nails and advises generally on foot care.

LEARNING POINTS FROM CASE HISTORY

- ○ **Older people may present late, often willing to put up with moderate to severe disability and handicap.**
- ○ **Mobility problems in older people are often multifactorial.**
- ○ **Simple interventions can often bring about significant improvements in mobility.**
- ○ **Older people with poor mobility require multi-professional input both in primary care and secondary care settings.**
- ○ **Sedative medication can exacerbate problems with mobility.**

Tutorial — mobility problems

Introduction

Ageing is associated with various kinds of deterioration and decline. Muscles become weaker, joints less flexible, and individuals tire more easily. Four out of ten people aged 50 years and over are sedentary, and more than half of over-50s and two-thirds of over-70s believe that they are doing enough exercise to keep fit. As a result, one-third of people over aged 70 cannot walk one-quarter of a mile on their own. By the age of 75, 22% are housebound and by 85 this has increased to 52.9%. Poor housing, poor social class, gender, age and visual problems all contribute to lack of exercise, exacerbated by the powerful negative effect of ageism. Those aged over 65 often report some kind of health and functional impairment. Presentation of disability is often silent and occult. The only way a GP may learn about this is through a request for a home visit because a patient is housebound.

Arthritis/rheumatism was the most common reported cause of chronic illness in the older population in the General Household Survey 1998. Similarly, diseases or complaints of the musculoskeletal system were reported in 26% of older patients aged over 65. As a result, older people with these conditions experience a range of problems including difficulty with walking, climbing stairs and bathing. Therefore, they require support from family, friends and neighbours and/or social services.

In the population of older women between the ages of 75 and 84, 48.5% reported that they had painful knees; back pain and painful feet were also common complaints. Foot problems increase with old age. A reported 65% of people over 85 cannot cut their own toenails, and less than half reported seeing a chiropodist in the last six months (OPCS 1996).

Osteoporosis is a risk factor for fractures. Osteoporotic fractures are associated with serious disabilities. Following a hip fracture, half the survivors cannot walk independently. Osteoporosis can also present with sudden onset of severe back pain resulting from fractures of the lumbar or thoracic spine.

Musculoskeletal disorders are not the only causes of poor mobility. Any acute or chronic illness can lead to reduced mobility and falls. Whatever the cause of poor mobility, it is important to diagnose any underlying illness, as well as start mobilisation as soon as that illness has resolved or started to improve.

In this tutorial we will examine three common causes of mobility problems in the elderly: osteoarthritis, polymyalgia rheumatica and gait disorders. A fourth cause, Parkinson's disease is dealt with in Chapter 5.

Common causes of impaired mobility in older people

Any acute or chronic illness can adversely affect mobility in older people. However, we will focus here on musculoskeletal problems.

OSTEOARTHRITIS

Osteoarthritis is a chronic degenerative joint disease that primarily affects weight-bearing joints. It is one of the most prevalent chronic conditions affecting the UK population and is a leading cause of disability amongst people aged 65 and over.

The joint instability, stiffness and muscle atrophy lead to decreased range of motion. Secondary inflammation related to osteoarthritis contributes to the two most dominant symptoms of pain and functional disability. The primary goals in the medical management of osteoarthritis are to minimise pain and maintain function. This is achieved through the use of medications, physical therapy, exercise, pain management and rest. Therapeutic exercise for osteoarthritis includes a range of motion, strengthening and flexibility exercises, as well as low impact aerobic and aquatic exercises.

Osteoarthritis is defined as pathological focal loss of articular cartilage with subchondral bone reaction. By the age of 70, 30% of women and 20% of men suffer from osteoarthritis of the knee, whereas only 15% of women and 10% of men in the same age group suffer from osteoarthritis of the hip. Risk factors for osteoarthritis of the knees are obesity and injury. The presence of an effusion and detectable warmth can often predict faster progression. Muscle wasting and weakness secondary to pain reduces function. Muscle ageing and loss of muscle mass in association with osteoarthritic joints give rise to increasing loss of function. Older people will experience increasing problems walking, climbing stairs and putting on socks and shoes. Osteoarthritis of the hip can present with pain in the groin or referred pain in the knee. Osteoarthritis of the knee can present with pain, swelling and (later on) instability giving rise to falls.

The patient's condition may well be compounded by depression, isolation and pain. The vicious cycle of pain, depression and demoralisation requires patience from both the GP and the specialist. Every patient's attendance should be regarded as an educational opportunity. The role of both a specialist and the GP is to ease pain, as well as consider opportunities to modify diet and to prescribe exercise. There is considerable evidence to show that quadriceps exercises for the knees (Petrella & Bartha 2000) improve the outcome for osteoarthritis of the knee.

Low back pain
Low back pain, which can and often does lead to mobility problems, is very common in old age and can respond to mobilisation and physiotherapy, just as it does in younger people. Some patients may present with low back pain on exercise due to spinal cord claudication. Others may present with unilateral or bilateral buttock pain caused by facet joint arthritis.

Physiotherapy can reduce pain in some cases, and occupational therapy can be useful in order to give advice on techniques to reduce pain on weight bearing and dressing. Some patients respond to local epidural injections or steroid injections into the facet joints. TENS machines may sometimes help. Patients can either buy them or physiotherapists may be able to loan them.

Role of the multidisciplinary team in the management
of osteoarthritis
Involvement of the multidisciplinary team in the management of osteoarthritis can be extremely helpful:

○ to confirm the diagnosis
○ to rule out other causes of arthritis
○ to give advice about the use of nonsteroidal anti-inflammatory drugs
○ to refer for X-ray and other imaging
○ to involve physiotherapists and occupational therapists
○ to give advice about changes to the home
○ to advise on footwear
○ to provide appropriate walking aids
○ to give advice on which exercises to use

○ to give advice on diet and weight loss when appropriate

○ to look for signs of associated psychological problems and offer help as appropriate.

In addition, the team has a duty to help patients manage their own disease. All health professionals should listen to the patient and should not trivialise the problem or underestimate the pain. The aim is to enable the patient to cope. Where medication is used, it should involve using the least harmful drug in the smallest effective dose. Home visits by the physiotherapist and the occupational therapist will help focus advice in the patient's everyday surroundings.

Medical treatment for osteoarthritis

A simple analgesic, such as paracetamol, is the drug of first choice. In the right dosage, this is effective and safe. Nonsteroidal anti-inflammatory drugs (NSAIDs) do have a place for short-term use but can cause side-effects (especially gastrointestinal), and there is some evidence to suggest that they may accelerate the progression of osteoarthritis. Cox II inhibitors have been suggested to be less likely to produce symptomatic ulcers, in comparison with nonsteroidals. However, the evidence for this is controversial, and there are also concerns about possible cardiovascular risks associated with these drugs. The use of chondroitin sulphate and glucosamine preparations has been shown in some studies to have benefit, and more recently sodium hyaluronidate injections into the knees for three to five weeks has been shown to produce some reduction in pain.

The role of surgery in osteoarthritis treatment

If the conservative measures discussed above have not been effective in significantly reducing the pain of osteoarthritis, referral to an orthopaedic surgeon is appropriate. Possible surgical interventions for osteoarthritis include joint injections, arthroscopic procedures (e.g. joint debridement, arthrodesis, osteotomy, arthroplasty and joint replacement).

The role of exercise and other activities in osteoarthritis management

The consequences of osteoarthritis are complex, as a decline in physical function may also have major psychosocial effects. Older people may experience a diminished sense of personal capability and self-esteem, which leads to a lifestyle which can become increasingly characterised by immobility, dependency and compromised well-being.

There is considerable evidence to show that a healthy lifestyle reduces disability levels and improves quality of life. Physiotherapy can reduce pain in some cases, and occupational therapy can be useful in order to give advice on techniques to reduce pain on weight bearing and dressing. Simple exercise, such as walking or swimming, can help maintain joint mobility. Recently, tai chi has been shown to enhance quality of life and functional mobility among older adults with osteoarthritis (Hartman et al 2000). It is thought that tai chi training is a safe and effective complementary therapy in the medical management of lower extremity osteoarthritis. Tai chi exercises include a series of gentle fluid movements, which are reputedly good for maintaining mobility and flexibility of the musculoskeletal system. There is some evidence that it does improve fitness outcomes, muscular strength, flexibility and percentage of body fat, as well as reducing the risk of falls in older people.

POLYMYALGIA RHEUMATICA (PMR)

The diagnosis of PMR should be suspected in any older person presenting with at least one month's history of persistent pain and stiffness in the neck, shoulder girdle or pelvic girdle. Characteristically, patients with polymyalgia rheumatica have bilateral discomfort involving the proximal limb and joint areas. The symptoms may be worse in the morning and will last for a minimum of 30 minutes. The pain worsens with movement and can interfere with activities of daily living.

Examination will usually reveal limitation of active and passive movements of the shoulders. Shoulder pain is the presenting finding in the majority of patients; hips and neck are less frequently involved. Systemic symptoms and signs are present in approximately one-third of patients and can include fever, malaise or fatigue, anorexia and weight loss. The diagnosis is usually made within 2–3 months of onset. An erythrocyte sedimentation rate (ESR) of at least 40 mm/hour is considered an essential diagnostic finding. Occasionally, some patients with polymyalgia rheumatica have been reported as having a normal sedimentation rate. The C-reactive protein has been found to be a more sensitive indicator of disease activity.

Corticosteroids are the drug of choice to treat PMR. An initial dose of 20 mg daily is adequate in most cases. Resolution of symptoms with steroid treatment is rapid, and most of the presenting problems will resolve over a few days. Steroid dosage can then be very gradually reduced over several months, depending on response. Regular reassessment of symptoms, ESR and/or the C-reactive protein are the most valuable methods of monitoring the disease. In older people, a treatment course of two years is often required. In a small minority of patients, long-term steroid therapy may be necessary. Calcium and vitamin D supplements should be given with corticosteroid therapy in all patients with polymyalgia rheumatica. In some patients, bisphosphonate therapy will be necessary.

GAIT DISORDERS

Independence in old age is governed not least by the ability to stand up, to walk, to turn and to lean. Timed walks and timed 'get up and go' from the sitting position are all predictors of the ability to perform activities of daily living, as well as the likelihood of being admitted to a nursing home or dying. The successful coordination of sensation, musculoskeletal function, motor control and attention will result in walking without assistance.

Normal older people will walk more slowly and will take shorter steps. The body position only changes slightly with age, unless diseases such as osteoporosis, kyphosis or Parkinson's disease are present. Many gait disorders are caused by either musculoskeletal problems or neurological disorders, or a combination of both (Box 4.1).

BOX 4.1: Gait disorders: remember to consider

- Tumours of the forebrain
- Subdural haematomas
- Cervical myelopathy
- Spinal cord claudication
- Drugs: alcohol, neuroleptics hypotensives, benzodiazepines
- Osteoarthritis of the knee and hips
- Vitamin D deficiency

Cerebellar or frontal lobe disorders will cause a breakdown in the motor control of gait. Frontal gait disorders, or gait apraxia, presenting with marche à petit pas (small shuffling steps) or magnetic gait (difficulty picking the feet off the floor) are caused by ischaemic damage to the periventricular white matter (shown on CT scan). These are common causes of difficulty in walking. Disturbances of the cerebellum impair posture and locomotion, producing ataxia, spasticity, dystonia and chorea. Parkinson's disease may initially produce mild symptoms but can progress into a much more widespread neurological disease (Chapter 5).

In any older patient with difficulties in walking, cervical myelopathy, B_{12} deficiency and progressive sensory loss should be considered. Claudication of the cauda equina caused by arthritis of the lumbar and sacral spine is an important and common condition which is characterised by the onset of severe pain, numbness and weakness in one or both legs. Exercise makes the patient lean forward, often mimicking vascular claudication, and is described as 'spinal cord claudication'. Patients are often described as walking like a crab.

Cervical myelopathy presents with an acute or slowly progressive spastic paraparesis. Initially, patients may complain of tingling with weakness of the hands, and later they develop stiffness and clumsiness of the legs. They have lower motor neurone signs at the site of the lesion, such as loss of reflexes, and below the level of the lesion they will have increased reflexes (i.e. hyporeflexia in the upper extremities and hyperreflexia in the lower extremities).

Older people with osteomalacia may develop proximal muscle weakness, leading to a waddling type of gait. It is more common to find sub-clinical levels of vitamin D in this age group, giving rise to muscle weakness particularly in those who are housebound or who come from the Indian subcontinent. Lack of exposure to sunlight is a potent cause of vitamin D deficiency.

KEY LEARNING POINTS — MOBILITY

○ With age there are changes in muscles and joints that can affect gait and predispose an older person to developing reduced mobility.

○ Exercise, and in particular tai chi, can not only improve muscle strength and mobility but also reduce the risk of falling.

○ An acute illness, such as pneumonia or urinary tract infection, can lead to poor mobility or immobility.

○ It is important to diagnose the exact cause of reduced mobility/immobility, as the correct management is dependent upon this.

○ Mobilisation should begin as soon as the acute phase of illness has resolved or started to improve.

○ The emotional consequences of long-term arthritic pain are considerable and should be addressed.

Reference

OPCS 1996, Living in Britain: Results from the 1994 General Household Survey, London HMSO.

Further reading

Hartman CA, Manos TM, Winter C. Effects of t'ai chi training on function and quality of life indicators in older adults with osteoarthritis. J Am Geriatrics Soc 2000; 48(12):1553–9.

Petrella RJ, Bartha C J. Home based exercise for older patients with knee arthritis: a randomised clinical trial. Rheumatology 2000; 27(9):2215–21.

Office for National Statistics. Living in Britain: Results from the 1998 General Household Survey, Stationery Office, London 2000.

Further information

Arthritis Care. **http://www.arthritiscare.org.uk.**

CHAPTER 5

The older patient with Parkinson's disease

CASE HISTORY

Mr. PD is 79 years old and was first diagnosed with Parkinson's disease when he was aged 71. At that time he presented to his GP complaining mainly of fatigue. The GP noticed the characteristic facial appearance and tremor of Parkinson's, and referred him to the neurology department. He has attended the neurologist at the local hospital every six months, seeing a variety of different trainee doctors and occasionally the consultant.

In the spring he notices that his walking has deteriorated. His wife is having to help him dress, and he is able to do little for himself. Mr. PD goes to the hospital and sees the specialist, who thinks that in addition to the Sinemet he is taking he should be started on a pramipexole (a dopamine agonist). The dosage is gradually increased. Initially, his walking improves but then his wife notices he is becoming confused. She is distraught when he tells her he is seeing strange animals on the floor and then accuses her of having an affair with the next door neighbour!

The GP is aware that the local hospital runs a Parkinson's disease clinic, led by a consultant geriatrician and coordinated by a specialist nurse. He phones up the neurologist and suggests that as Mr. PD is getting older and is starting to develop multiple problems he would like to refer him to the clinic. The neurologist agrees this is a good plan. The Parkinson's disease clinic is held weekly in the day hospital, with access to physiotherapists, occupational therapists and speech therapists. When he attends the clinic, Mr. PD sees the consultant who undertakes a Parkinson's Disease Rating Scale, a mini mental state and a geriatric depression scale. The specialist also completes a full physical examination and arranges for the nurse to measure Mr. PD's timed 'up and go' and a timed six-metre walk.

Following this examination the consultant geriatrician organises a CT scan of the brain, ECG and chest X-ray, as well as routine blood tests to rule out any other significant pathology.

Mr. PD confides to the staff that not only is he having problems getting about and is seeing strange things, but he is also having increasing difficulties swallowing.

He is seen by the speech therapist who identifies his problems with swallowing and recommends that he receives a pureed diet and thickened fluids to prevent aspiration.

His dopamine agonist is reduced and he is given a period of intense physiotherapy. He is seen by the occupational therapist, who visits him at home and makes some adaptations to his flat. The investigations do not show any abnormalities. He is found to be depressed. The consultant starts him on Donepezil, as there is some evidence that anticholinesterase inhibitors may prevent and/or reduce the neuropsychiatric side-effects of treatment. She also reduces his pramipexole to the minimum therapeutic dose.

Mr. PD is also noted to have postural hypotension on standing . This is a common side-effect not only of the disease but of the medication. He is then given advice about how he should rise from both beds and chairs. He is also encouraged to wear support stockings. After a few weeks, he and his wife are pleased that his hallucinations have gone and that at the same time his mobility is improving.

The role of the hospital team in management of Parkinson's disease

○ To consider further investigations, to rule out secondary causes of Parkinson's Disease.

○ To do a full neurological examination, including tests for gait and bradykinesia, brief assessment scales, Parkinson's Disease Rating Scale/Webster scores, 6–12 m walks, timed 'up and go'.

○ To confirm whether the patient has a response to dopa by doing assessments before and after the introduction of the levodopa.

○ To reduce patient's distress, to control symptoms and to improve prognosis.

○ To prevent complications of treatment.

○ To stage Parkinson's disease.

○ To educate patient and family and carers.

LEARNING POINTS FROM THE CASE HISTORY

● **Parkinson's disease is a progressive disease with needs of individual changing with time.**

● **In addition to drug therapy individuals will require input from every professional member of the multidisciplinary team.**

Tutorial — Parkinson's disease (PD)

Parkinson's disease has a prevalence of 1% in the population aged over 65 and is the second most common neurodegenerative disease in old age. The goal of drug treatment is to manage the disease by reducing disability, such that the impact on both the patient and carer(s) is minimised. Although prevalence of Parkinson's disease is high, incidence is low, and general practitioners will see only a few new cases. Misdiagnosis of the condition in the early stages may result in prolonged symptoms and inappropriate drug treatment, as well as the possibility of a long wait to see a neurologist.

Recent evidence shows that only 17.3% of the variation in health-related quality of life in patients suffering from Parkinson's disease could be explained by the severity of the disease. It appears that good communication skills provided with effective counselling and behavioural modification improved the outcome of treatment. Specialist nurses have also been shown to improve well-being.

It is recommended that like most people with chronic neurological disorders, patients with PD need to be looked after by a multidisciplinary team which includes a general practitioner, a neurologist or a geriatrician with interest in PD, pharmacist, specialist nurse, physiotherapist, occupational therapist and speech therapist. The global declaration of Mumbai (Parkinson's Disease Charter) describes the general approach which should be provided for any patient with PD:

○ Be referred to a doctor with a special interest in Parkinson's disease.
○ Receive an accurate diagnosis.

○ Have access to support services.

○ Receive continuous care.

○ Take part in managing the illness.

The classic symptoms and signs of Parkinson's disease are:

○ Tremor — most marked at rest and often described as 'pill rolling'.

○ Bradykinesia — slow movement, monotonous speech, expressionless face, decreased blink rate, micrographia.

○ Rigidity — limbs resist passive extension and may judder because of coexistent tremor to produce 'cogwheel rigidity'.

○ Postural instability — short shuffling steps with flexed trunk (festinant gait).

There are no definitive diagnostic tests available. Clinical history and examination supplemented by tests to rule out other causes of Parkinsonism form the basis of diagnosis. Many other diseases in old age can cause parkinsonism (Box 5.1), and treatment should not be started until other causes have been ruled out.

BOX 5.1: Diseases mimicking Parkinson's disease

- Cerebrovascular disease (present acutely)
- Neuroleptic drugs
- Parkinson's plus
- Steele–Richardson syndrome
- Multi-system atrophy
- Benign tremor
- Lewy body dementia
- Cerebral tumours
- Head trauma

In the sixties before the introduction of levodopa and its successors, Hoehn and Yahr classified the disease in terms of the following rating scale:

Stage I   Unilateral symptoms

Stage II   Bilateral mild disease

Stage III   Loss of balance

Stage IV   Unable to live independently

Stage V   Confined to a wheelchair.

Medical treatment of Parkinson's disease in older people

Levodopa is the initial treatment of choice in old age. The use of anticholinergics is not encouraged because of severe side-effects. A test dose of levodopa may be given in the clinic, or a 2-week course of combined levodopa and dopa decarboxylase (enzyme inhibitor) can be given. In order to assess effect of therapy it is useful to take a baseline measure of functional disability before treatment and repeat any test after the initial trial. Measurement of timed 'up and go' (Box 5.2) and Webster's Parkinson's Disease Rating Scale (Appendix 3, p. 234) are useful tools in this respect. It is only beneficial to continue treatment if patients are showing evidence of positive response.

BOX 5.2: Timed 'up and go' test

The timed 'up and go' test measures, in seconds, the time taken by a patient to stand up from a standard arm chair (approximate seat height of 46 cm, arm height 65 cm), walk a distance of 3 metres, turn, walk back to the chair and sit down again. The patient wears their regular footwear and uses any usual walking aid (none, stick or frame).

> **BOX 5.2:** Timed 'up and go' test—continued
>
> No physical assistance is given. They start with their back against the chair, their arms resting on the arm rests and their walking aid at hand. They are instructed—on the word 'go'—to get up and walk at a comfortable and safe pace to a line on the floor 3 metres away, turn, return to the chair and sit down again. The subject walks through the test once before being timed, in order to become familiar with the test. Either a wristwatch with a second hand or a stopwatch can be used to time the performance.

CARBIDOPA-LEVODOPA AND LEVODOPA/BENSERAZIDE HYDROCHLORIDE (CO-BENELDOPA)

The combination of carbidopa-levodopa and levodopa/benserazide hydrochloride (co-beneldopa) has revolutionised the treatment of Parkinson's disease. Levodopa still remains the gold standard for management. Those with rigidity and bradykinesia generally respond best. Tremor may be difficult to suppress.

MAO AND COMT INHIBITORS

Inhibitors of MAO or COMT enhance and prolong its effect and are thereby dopa-sparing. Direct agonists used alone may avoid long-term levodopa-related treatment problems but usually need to be combined with levodopa in due course for satisfactory control.

MAO INHIBITOR (SELEGILINE)

This monoamine oxidase inhibitor (Type B) was thought to slow the progress of Parkinson's disease if used from first diagnosis. However, one study showed an unexpectedly high mortality with combined levodopa/selegiline therapy after three years, possibly due to autonomic side-effects. It still has a role in early and late Parkinson's disease, but its place should remain under scrutiny, and should be slowly reduced and stopped if confusion, falls or hypotension occurs. Zelapar is a recently introduced buccal melt preparation — the dose is 1.25 mg rather than 5–10 mg of the oral preparations.

COMT INHIBITOR (ENTACAPONE)

This inhibitor of the alternative pathway for dopamine break-down can smooth out fluctuations and permit a reduction of levodopa dose (typically by 30–50%).

DOPAMINE AGONISTS (BROMOCRIPTINE, PERGOLIDE, ROPINIROLE, CABERGOLINE, PRAMIPEXOLE, APOMORPHINE)

These can be used either as monotherapy or in addition to levodopa. It is thought that early monotherapy with dopamine agonists may be neuroprotective and thus prevent some of the later complications. The perception that the clinical response is less than with levodopa, with a higher incidence of side-effects, has been challenged by recent trial findings.

AMANTADINE

This drug is occasionally used in the later stages and has some dopamine agonist effect.

General points about Parkinson's disease

Once the diagnosis and management plan have been established, the primary care team should watch out for complications and establish relationships with specialist P.D. nurses. Ensures that there is rapid access for the patient if the symptoms and signs change.

Treatment at this stage should relieve symptoms, improve function, prevent complications and maintain mood and good health. The patient may have concerns about driving, inheritance of the disease, finance, disability allowances and sexual relationships.

Disease progression

After 5 years, 30–80% of patients experience end-of-dose deterioration in mobility. They can also experience problems with dyskinesias, which are involuntary movements of the head and neck as well as facial grimaces. The dyskinesias will usually occur at peak dose levels of levodopa, but dysphasic dyskinesias can occur at peak doses and low doses of medication.

Speech disturbances can occur in about 60–70% of parkinsonian patients, whilst 40–60% of patients experience dysphagia. Autonomic disturbances are a significant problem in more advanced Parkinson's, and 60% of patients will experience constipation caused by prolonged transit time in the gut exacerbated by inadequate fluid intake. Autonomic failure will also cause erectile dysfunction in 40–60%. Patients may develop urinary frequency and urgency, leading onto urinary incontinence.

Orthostatic hypotension occurs in 10–20% of sufferers and will exacerbate postural instability. Drenching sweats at the end of off-periods are a function of fluctuations in levodopa levels.

Sleep disorders are common. Insomnia is thought to be secondary to a difficulty in sleep initiation and can also be exacerbated by problems of turning in bed at night and depression, nightmares and urinary frequency.

Early treatment of PD is concentrated on the management of bradykinesia, while treatment of advanced disease is concerned with management of motor fluctuations. The presence of late complications in Parkinson's disease is increasing (Box 5.3), and severe disability is reported in 53% of Parkinson's disease 4 years after treatment is initiated.

BOX 5.3: Late complications of Parkinson's disease

- Motor fluctuations
- Falling
- Bulbar abnormalities
- Autonomic disturbances
- Psychiatric disturbances or disorders
- Feet abnormalities
- Cognitive dysfunction
- Dyskinesias
- Pain

If there is an acute deterioration in signs and symptoms, it is important to look for other diseases (e.g. infections). Remember to check for signs of subdural haematoma in patients who may have fallen.

Psychiatric/neuropsychiatric problems

As the disease progresses, psychiatric manifestations occur with greater frequency (Box 5.4). Parkinson's disease is now regarded as a neuropsychiatric/neurodegenerative condition, with a high prevalence of depression and dementia. Dementia occurs in 30–40% of older people with Parkinson's disease, and similarly 30–40% of patients with Parkinson's disease suffer from depression. Sinemet and Madopar, as well as dopamine agonists, can exacerbate psychoses including hallucinations and delusions. Sometimes a consultant in old age psychiatry may have to work closely with the specialist team. In addition to the more complex psychiatric conditions, anxiety and depression are common. Psychologists can provide significant help to an older person with such a worrying disease.

BOX 5.4: Psychiatric symptoms associated with Parkinson's disease

- Depression/mania
- Dementia
- Anxiety
- Sleep disorders
- Sexual dysfunction
- Hallucinations with preserved insight
- Medication-induced psychotic disorders
- Delirium
- Schizophrenic-like psychotic disorder

Bladder symptoms

Detrusor instability or urgency of urine can be present in 50–70% of patients and may be exacerbated by constipation, dehydration and cognitive impairment. Patients may not necessarily respond to the traditional medication for detrusor instability because the anticholinergic drugs will tend to exacerbate postural instability and falls. Other methods should be considered for the management of these unpleasant symptoms.

Other diseases and Parkinson's disease

PD is most common in old age, and older people tend to have other medical problems which may require attention and treatment. The GP and old age medicine specialists are in the best position to monitor and manage any co-morbidity and can always seek specialist advice when another illness affects Parkinson's control. For example, the most common problems in all older people are cardiovascular and cerebrovascular diseases, and treatment of these may exacerbate the side-effects experienced with the drugs used for PD (e.g. postural hypotension).

Voluntary organisations, such as the Parkinson's Disease Society, play an important role in supporting patients and carers, not only by providing advice and welfare but also by being a source of information and literature about the disease.

The role of surgery in Parkinson's disease

With improvements in neurosurgical techniques and neuro-imaging in recent years, there has been a great deal of interest in the potential value of surgery for Parkinson's disease.

Surgical techniques which have been tried for Parkinson's disease include:

○ thalamotomy

○ pallidotomy

○ deep brain stimulation

○ striatal grafting of dopaminergic fetal tissue.

Over the last few years, a number of groups has reported some encouraging results for surgery in patients with severe

Parkinson's disease, but these have in general been younger people. The evidence for benefit over risk in the elderly Parkinson's population is not good.

KEY LEARNING POINTS— PARKINSON'S DISEASE

○ True Parkinson's disease must be distinguished from parkinsonism, symptoms of which do not respond to medical treatment with levodopa.

○ Gait disturbances are common in patients with Parkinson's disease.

○ As the disease progresses, the needs of individuals change. Regular follow-up is essential, not only to monitor the progression of disease but to monitor side-effects of drug therapy.

○ With progression of disease, individuals may experience end-of-dose effect, speech problems, dysphagia, autonomic disturbances (including postural hypotension), sleep problems and neuropsychiatric disturbances.

○ Drugs are not the only treatment—older patients with Parkinson's disease require input from each professional member of the multidisciplinary team in the primary and secondary care settings.

References

Bhatia K, Brook DJ, et al. Guidelines for the management of Parkinson's disease. The Parkinson's Disease Consensus Working Group. Hosp Med 1998; 59(6):469–480.

Kale R, Menken M. Who should look after people with Parkinson's disease? BMJ 2004; 328:62–63.

Further reading

Beers MH, Berkow R. (eds.) The Merck manual of geriatrics. 3rd ed. Whitehouse Station, NJ: Merck Research Laboratories; 2000.

Howse K, Prophet H. Improving the health of older Londoners : reviewing the evidence. Centre for Policy on Ageing; 2000.

Further information

Parkinson's Disease Society **http://www.parkinsons.org.uk.** Helpline Freephone: 0800 800 0303

European Parkinson's Disease Association. **www.epda.eu.com.** Association produces a series of useful information leaflets for people with Parkinson's, their families, and healthcare professionals.

CHAPTER 6

The older patient with breathing problems

Mr. BA is 83 years old. Until recently he has been active and independent. However, over the last month he has been getting short of breath more easily and now finds that when he goes out to walk his dog he has to rest every few yards to catch his breath. He initially put this down to old age but during the last two nights he has had quite severe breathlessness during the night and so he has decided to visit his GP and ask for something to help his breathing.

The GP can see straight away that Mr. BA is breathless, even after walking the few yards from the waiting room. He goes through the patient's history. He hears about his increasing breathlessness on exertion which is now also present when lying down. Mr. BA has not had any chest pain but does have quite swollen ankles. He has not had a cough and is not bringing up any phlegm. Mr. BA used to smoke but gave up several years ago after a bad chest infection. He is taking bendroflumethiazide for his blood pressure and the occasional ibuprofen when his back is playing up. On examination, the GP finds Mr. BA to be well-orientated with good short-term memory. He is breathless at rest with a pulse of 120 beats per minute and a respiratory rate of 25 per minute. There are fine inspiratory crackles in both lungs at the back. His blood pressure is 150/90. His JVP is elevated almost to his ear lobes, and both his ankles are swollen with pitting oedema. His liver is also enlarged.

The GP diagnoses acute heart failure and explains to Mr. BA that he needs to go to hospital for immediate treatment. He agrees with this and telephones his family to explain the situation.

On arrival at A&E, he is seen by the duty registrar who confirms the GP's findings and arranges for him to have a series of investigations. The results are as follows: his chest X-ray shows pulmonary vascular congestion and cardiomegaly and his ECG reveals a sinus tachycardia with left ventricular hypertrophy and an old inferior infarct. His haemoglobin is normal but his urea is slightly elevated, and his LFTs show a raised alkaline phosphatase. An echocardiogram shows an ejection fraction of 35% with some mitral incompetence. A diagnosis of heart failure secondary to coronary heart disease is made, and he is treated with intravenous nitrates initially and then with intravenous diuretics to reduce his fluid overload. His ibuprofen is stopped and he is placed on an ACE inhibitor. He is put on a fluid input/output chart and daily weights. He has a rapid diuresis and over the following days his oedema resolves and he loses 6 kg in weight. He is started on oral loop diuretics and continued on his ACE inhibitors and, once stable, commenced on beta-blockers, as there are no contraindications.

After five days he is much better and is sent home with arrangements to be seen in outpatients in six weeks. He is also advised to see the GP for review and to make sure that he understands his diagnosis and treatment plan. With his permission, the ward nurse meets his daughter and explains to her what is going on with her father. Arrangements are also made for social services to assess his care needs at home.

CASE HISTORY 2

A GP looks after a 40-bedded nursing home. He is called in to see Mrs. BB, an 84-year-old lady with known COPD and early dementia. Mrs. BB is on three regular inhalers and is normally mobile and fairly independent. Recently, the staff have noticed that she has a bad cough, is not eating much and has a temperature of 37.5° C. The GP visits the home and examines the patient. He diagnoses an acute exacerbation of her COPD and starts her on amoxicillin 500 mg, three times a day. Two days later there is no improvement in Mrs. BB's condition, and the staff are worried about her. She is now not eating or drinking, her temperature has risen to 38.5° C and she doesn't want to get out of bed. They also notice that her blood pressure has dropped to 85/70 and her heart rate is 130. The GP returns to see Mrs. BB and finds her much worse. She is confused, unable to communicate and has a respiratory rate of 40, dullness at her right base with associated bronchial breathing and expiratory crackles. He discusses the situation with the staff and also her relatives. With their agreement, he organises for her immediate admission to hospital where his diagnosis of pneumonia is confirmed by chest X-ray. She is also noted to have a raised white count and ESR. She is treated with intravenous clarithromycin to which she make a good response. She is given intravenous fluids for dehydration and oxygen by nasal cannulae for her hypoxia. After 10 days she is well enough to return to the residential home.

LEARNING POINTS FROM CASE HISTORIES

- **Acute breathlessness in the elderly is usually cardiac or respiratory in origin.**
- **Elderly patients may often tolerate breathlessness for some time before presenting.**

- Elderly patients may deteriorate rapidly, and hospital investigation and treatment should not be delayed if symptoms do not improve following initial management at home.
- Given the many possible causes of breathlessness, a systematic approach to diagnosis is essential.
- Assessment should always take into account the patient's previous history.
- Careful history and examination will usually lead to correct diagnosis.

Tutorial — breathlessness in the elderly

Breathlessness or dyspnoea is a feeling of difficulty or laboured breathing that is out of proportion to the patient's level of physical activity. The experience of dyspnoea depends on its severity and its underlying pulmonary or cardiac cause. Older patients present special difficulties in terms of diagnosis as several causes of breathlessness often coexist. There is also evidence that they may experience a reduced perception of their respiratory problems which may delay their seeking help. Also they tend to attribute symptoms to ageing or general de-conditioning, which may further delay correct diagnosis and adequate therapy. This chapter concentrates on breathlessness arising from the two most common and important causes in the elderly: heart failure and chronic obstructive pulmonary disease (COPD). However, it is always important when assessing breathless patients to be aware of other possible causes (Table 6.1).

The following broad categories cover most of the common causes of breathlessness:

○ cardiac

○ respiratory

○ neuromuscular

○ haematological

○ metabolic and endocrine

○ renal failure

○ others, e.g. trauma, obesity, poor fitness, anxiety and panic attacks.

The gradual onset of breathlessness secondary to either heart failure or COPD will lead to a progressive inability to perform activities of daily living. It is important to take a careful history, encouraging the patient to describe the nature and progression

Table 6.1: Causes of acute and chronic breathlessness

Acute breathlessness	Chronic breathlessness
• Myocardial infarction • Disturbances of the heart rhythm • Left ventricular failure • Pleural effusion • Pulmonary fibrosis • Lung cancer • Pulmonary embolism • Pneumonia • Acute exacerbation of COPD • Asthma • Pneumothorax • Anaphylactic shock • Airway obstruction (e.g. inhaled foreign body) • Anxiety/hyperventilation • Chest injuries, e.g. fractured ribs	• Ischaemic heart disease • Left ventricular dysfunction • Chronic obstructive pulmonary disease (COPD) • Pulmonary hypertension • Asthma • Pulmonary fibrosis • Lung cancer • Muscular disorders (e.g. myasthenia gravis) • Anaemia • Hypothyroidism • Hyperthyroidism • Anxiety • Poor fitness • Deformities of the chest • Obesity

of their breathing problems in these terms. The New York Heart Association (NYHA) classification for heart failure (Table 6.2) and the Medical Research Council (MRC) grading for COPD record very similar hierarchies of symptoms and can help the clinician define the cause and rate of progression of the disease.

Acute breathlessness

Dyspnoea is defined as acute when it appears suddenly or within at most a few hours in a patient who has not previously

Table 6.2: New York Heart Association (NYHA) classification of heart failure

Grade 1	No symptoms, no limitation
Grade 2	Mild symptoms with slight limitations during ordinary activity but comfortable at rest
Grade 3	Marked limitations in function with symptoms even during less ordinary activities; comfortable only at night
Grade 4	Severe limitations even while at rest

complained of shortness of breath. Diagnosis can generally be made from additional features of the history and examination. It may be difficult because some older people with acute myocardial infarction do not present with acute central chest pain, and some elderly with pneumonia may not have fever or a raised white cell count.

Chronic breathlessness

Dyspnoea may worsen slowly over months or even years before a patient seeks medical advice. The occurrence of chronic dyspnoea increases with age, as the prevalence of its two most important causes (chronic heart failure and COPD) also increase with age. The most successful approach to diagnosis is to focus on the circumstances surrounding breathlessness and the timing of its occurrence.

Heart failure in the elderly

Heart failure is a complex clinical syndrome which can result from any structural or functional cardiac disorder which impairs the ability of the ventricles to fill with or eject blood.

The cardinal manifestations are dyspnoea/shortness of breath and fatigue, which limit exercise tolerance and cause fluid retention. Fluid retention in turn may cause pulmonary congestion and peripheral oedema. Pulmonary congestion will lead to shortness of breath. Heart failure is now the preferred title rather than the older phrase of congestive cardiac failure.

Heart failure is common. It has an incidence of 20–30 per 1000 per year. Significantly, its prevalence increases with age, and in those aged over 80, 30% have heart failure. It is a major problem for the NHS, consuming 1–2% of health care costs, 70% of which relate to hospitalisations which can be recurrent and prolonged. It has been shown that it is responsible for 5% of medical emergencies, and in primary care most people with this diagnosis will be seen 11–14 times/year.

As a condition, heart failure is associated with a significant morbidity and mortality. Irrespective of age, men and women have an almost equal (20%) likelihood of developing heart failure over a lifetime. Mortality in recent times remains high at 40% dying within a year of a new diagnosis. Mortality then drops to 10% a year. Prognosis is rarely discussed with patients and carers/relatives, despite having a comparable prognosis to cancer. Clinical trials have been targeted at younger people, who more often have left ventricular dysfunction. Characteristically, symptoms fluctuate unrelated to medication, and there is a poor relationship between cardiac performance and symptoms. Diabetics and patients with atherosclerotic/peripheral vascular disease are more likely to develop progressive heart failure.

Unfortunately, recent studies have shown that in a primary care setting, 49% of patients with a diagnosis of heart failure had had an ECG, only 42% had an echocardiogram and only 54% were on appropriate medication. Better collaboration between primary and secondary care services for older people with heart failure will improve the treatment of these patients.

Heart failure on the whole is associated with a wide spectrum of left ventricular functional abnormalities. In diastolic heart failure there is an impairment of filling, and in systolic heart failure there is a dilated chamber with reduced wall movement/motion with preserved filling.

In some older people, there is a combination of systolic and diastolic dysfunction. An ejection fraction of less than 40% needs to be demonstrated on an echocardiogram to make the diagnosis of left ventricular dysfunction. For the diagnosis of diastolic dysfunction, there needs to be more than one index of impairment in ventricular filling.

Coronary heart disease is the cause in two-thirds of cases of left ventricular systolic dysfunction. Other causes include cardiomyopathy secondary to hypertension, thyroid disease, valvular disease, anaemia, alcoholism, myocarditis and idiopathic cardiomyopathy.

DIAGNOSIS OF HEART FAILURE

There is no single diagnostic test for heart failure. The diagnosis is made through careful history taking, physical examination and specific investigations. In addition to the normal history, it is important that the clinician considers and asks about any history of the following: hypertension, anaemia, diabetes, cholesterol, coronary and valvular heart disease, chest irradiation, drugs and alcohol. A careful examination including both cardiovascular and respiratory system is essential. The presence of right or left ventricular enlargement, an elevated JVP and a third heart sound are supportive of the diagnosis. The presence of volume overload will be detected by an elevated jugular venous pressure (JVP). There is evidence of an elevation of right-sided pressure in 86% of patients with elevated pressure due to left ventricular systolic dysfunction. Most of them will demonstrate volume overload and peripheral oedema, but some older people will have peripheral dependant oedema because of inactivity. In many cases, assuming the patient is well enough, basic investigation can take place in primary care. This should include FBC, U&E, glucose, lipids, LFTs, TFT, chest X-ray and ECG. More specialised tests, including echocardiography and beta-natriuretic peptide levels, may require referral to secondary care depending on local arrangements.

Cardiac disease should be suspected if there is evidence of a previous myocardial infarction, left ventricular hypertrophy or an arrhythmia. An echocardiogram demonstrating an ejection fraction of less than 40% confirms the presence of left ventricular dysfunction. MRI, CT scan or radionucleotide ventriculography can also be useful in particular cases.

TREATMENT OF HEART FAILURE

The goals of treatment of heart failure should be to enable the patient to adapt their lifestyle in order to remain as active as possible. Older people should be given a clear explanation about their condition. Patients may be more likely to be compliant with their treatment if the side-effects and effects of medications are made clear to them.

Once the nature and cause of heart failure has been defined, physicians should focus on the clinical assessment in terms of their functional capacity and the type, severity and duration of symptoms while performing activities of daily living. They should be encouraged to define what they want to do but can no longer do and to adapt their life style to maximise their independence. In the short-term but not in the long-term, exercise has been shown to improve capacity comparable with pharmacological interventions (Box 6.1).

The advantages of regular review are just beginning to be appreciated, and the appointment of specialist heart failure nurses to work with these patients is being encouraged by government.

BOX 6.1: NICE (2003) guidelines for the treatment of heart failure

The basis for a historical diagnosis of heart failure should be reviewed, and only patients whose diagnosis is confirmed should be managed in accordance with the guideline.

Doppler 2D echocardiographic examination should be performed to exclude important valve disease, assess the systolic (and diastolic) function of the left ventricle and detect intracardiac shunts.

All patients with heart failure due to left ventricular systolic dysfunction should be considered for treatment with an angiotensin-converting enzyme (ACE) inhibitor.

Beta-blockers licensed for heart failure should be initiated in patients with heart failure due to left ventricular systolic dysfunction after diuretic and ACE inhibitor therapy (regardless of whether or not symptoms persist after such therapy).

All patients with chronic heart failure require monitoring, which should include:

- clinical assessment of functional capacity, fluid status, cardiac rhythm, and cognitive and nutritional status
- review of medication, including need for changes and possible side-effects
- serum urea, electrolytes and creatinine.

> **BOX 6.1:** NICE (2003) guidelines for the treatment of heart failure — continued
>
> Patients with heart failure should generally be discharged from hospital only when their clinical condition is stable and the management plan is optimised.
>
> The primary care team, patient and carer must be aware of the management plan.
>
> Management of heart failure should be seen as a shared responsibility between patient and health care professional.

Drug treatment of heart failure

○ **Diuretics** tend to work rapidly to improve symptoms but should not be used alone. Loop diuretics act on the loop of Henle by increasing the sodium excretion by up to 20–25%, whereas thiazides and potassium-sparing drugs act on the distal portion of the renal tubule and only increase the sodium excretion by 5–10% of the filtered load.

○ **Angiotensin converting enzyme (ACE) inhibitors** work through the renin–angiotensin system by blocking the conversion of angiotensin-1 to angiotensin-2. In the long-term, they increase survival, alleviate symptoms and improve clinical status and wellbeing. It is recommended that they should be started at a low dose and be used initially with diuretics in cases of fluid overload. Renal function should be tested within two weeks. The most common side-effects are hypotension, dizziness and worsening renal function.

○ **Beta-blockers** work by inhibiting the adverse effects of the sympathetic nervous system. Bisoprolol, metoprolol, and carvedilol are recommended for their greater cardioselectivity but should only be used in stable heart failure when they can be introduced very slowly and in low doses. They are not recommended in older patients with a systolic pressure of below 110, or with slow heart rates of 60 or below.

○ **Digoxin** has been shown to increase survival and should be considered in those who are not responding well to ACE inhibitors and diuretics.

The following drugs have been shown to exacerbate symptoms of heart failure and should be avoided:

○ Antiarrhythmic drugs (only amiodarone has been shown not to adversely affect survival).

○ Calcium-channel blockers (only amlodipine does not affect survival).

○ Nonsteroidal drugs all cause sodium retention.

FOLLOW-UP IN OLDER PEOPLE WITH HEART FAILURE

The benefits of ongoing review have already been mentioned and can be provided by GP, specialist physician or a heart failure nurse. Patients should be regularly monitored for their symptoms, exercise tolerance and functional capacity. Their renal function will need to be regularly checked.

As heart failure progresses, there is a decline in renal perfusion which limits response to diuretic therapy. At that point, a second complementary diuretic such as bendroflumethiazide or metolazone can be introduced. Patients requiring intravenous diuretics and/or dopamine and dobutamine will need admission to hospital. Spironolactone is useful for those with preserved renal function and should be given in smaller dose in older people. As always, every effort should be made to devise an oral regimen that can match symptomatic improvement and reduce risk of deterioration. Older patients on large doses of diuretics and ACE inhibitors will need to have more regular monitoring of their renal function.

REFRACTORY END-STAGE HEART FAILURE AND PALLIATIVE CARE

Most older people with heart failure respond favourably to treatment, but some do not improve and will gradually deteriorate, developing symptoms on minimal exertion, with increasing difficulty carrying out activities of daily living.

Once the diagnosis has been reconfirmed and all therapeutic options have been explored, it may be necessary to accept that the patient is in refractory or end-stage cardiac failure. End-stage cardiac failure is a terminal illness and can involve considerable suffering for patients and their families. These patients require just as much attention to their palliative care needs as those dying of other incurable diseases, such as cancers. The most commonly reported distressing symptoms are:

○ dyspnoea

○ pain (often pain all over — non-specified cause)

○ overwhelming tiredness

○ functional impairment (difficulty walking)

○ depression

○ anxiety.

Much of their management can be served by the primary care team with support from specialists in secondary care. The palliative care approach should concentrate on quality of life and good symptom control, taking into account the needs of both patient and carers. It should be remembered that specialist palliative care teams are very able and willing to contribute to care of end-stage heart failure patients, especially in the following circumstances:

○ difficult symptom control

○ request to cease treatment

○ patients who wish to pursue non-aggressive/non-invasive management of end-stage disease

○ support for terminal care.

Acute respiratory causes of shortness of breath

The main respiratory causes of acute shortness of breath are pneumonia and acute exacerbation of COPD. The classic symptoms and signs of a lower respiratory tract infection, such as fever and cough, may not always be present in older people. Community acquired pneumonia, although common and often associated with a rapid deterioration, can be more difficult to diagnose in an older person. It should be strongly suspected if there is a sudden onset of confusion in a patient with a rapid respiratory rate with or without grunting respiration, abnormal added wheezes or expiratory crackles and a tachycardia.

INDICATIONS FOR ADMISSION TO HOSPITAL

○ Temperature over 37.8°C.

○ Heart rate over 100 beats/minute.

○ Respiratory rate over 24 breaths/minute.

○ Systolic blood pressure less than 90 mmHg.

○ Abnormal mental status and inability to take oral medication.

○ Inadequate support during illness at home.

Streptococcus pneumoniae remains the most important organism in community acquired pneumonia, even in patients with underlying COPD. Older patients with COPD who present with community acquired pneumonia usually have similar organisms to those with pneumonia.

Criteria for admission to hospital for patients with acute exacerbations of COPD are as follows:

○ marked increase in respiratory symptoms

○ severe COPD

○ onset of new physical signs

○ failure to respond to initial medical treatment

○ newly occurring arrhythmias or hypotension

○ confusion, and insufficient home support.

It has been shown that admission prevention schemes (such as hospital-at-home schemes, primary care liaison with a specialist respiratory nurse and intermediate care schemes) can all improve the care of these patients and reduce their need for admission to hospital.

INVESTIGATIONS IN ACUTE BREATHLESSNESS

Sometimes, investigation may be possible in primary care but more often this will take place on referral to secondary care in more severe cases. Chest X-ray, ECG, FBC, ESR, U&E, and C-reactive protein and arterial blood gases are all helpful in determining the cause and severity of the problem.

RECOMMENDATION FOR TREATMENT

Amoxicillin and/or clarithromycin are indicated as first-line treatments of untreated, non-severe community acquired chest infections.

Chronic obstructive pulmonary disease

Chronic obstructive pulmonary disease (COPD) is characterised by air flow limitation that is not fully reversible and is usually both regressive and associated with an abnormal inflammatory response of the lungs to noxious particles or gases. Breathlessness is the main symptom of COPD. This will increase as the condition deteriorates, and patients can enter a spiral of deterioration which often leads to social isolation, weight loss, deconditioning, immobilisation and depression.

A diagnosis of COPD should be considered in older patients who have smoked and who present with exertional breathlessness, chronic cough, regular sputum production, frequent winter bronchitis or wheeze. The presence of air flow obstruction should be confirmed by spirometry (Table 6.3). The patients themselves could be asked to scale their breathlessness by using the scale in Table 6.4.

DIAGNOSIS

A differential diagnosis between heart failure and COPD is fundamental to initiating the correct treatment. A diagnosis of COPD should be made on the basis of the Global Initiative in Obstructive Lung Disease and the NICE (National Institute for Clinical Excellence) guidelines. They define air flow obstruction as a ratio of less than 0.7 between forced expiratory volume in one second (FEV1) and forced vital capacity (FVC).

It is important to exclude asthma in any patient who presents with breathlessness. A careful history and examination should be taken. Special investigations should include spirometry. A chest X-ray is not helpful in a diagnosis but should be performed to exclude carcinoma of the bronchus in smokers. The

Table 6.3: Stages of chronic obstructive pulmonary disease (COPD)

Stages	COPD	Criteria
0	At risk	Normal spirometry, chronic symptoms (cough, sputum production)
1	Mild COPD	FEV1/FVC less than 70%, FEV1 greater than 80% predicted without chronic symptoms
2	Moderate	FEV1/FVC less than 70%; FEV1 ≥50% but less than 80% predicted
3	Severe	FEV1/FVC less than 70%; FEV1 ≥30% but less than 40% with or without symptoms
4	Very severe	FEV1 less than 30% predicted or less than 50% plus respiratory symptoms

Table 6.4: Patient self-rating scale for breathlessness

Please tick in the box that applies to you (one box only):

Box 1 ❑	I only get short of breath with strenuous exercise
Box 2 ❑	I get short of breath when hurrying on the level or walking up a slight incline
Box 3 ❑	I walk slower than people of the same age on the level because of breathlessness or I have to stop for breath when walking at my own pace on the level
Box 4 ❑	I stop for breath after walking about 100 yards or after a few minutes on the level
Box 5 ❑	I am too breathless to leave the house or I am breathless when dressing or undressing

Table 6.5: Approaches to the management of COPD

Stop smoking	This is the most important measure in preventing disease progression
Inhaler device	The appropriate inhaler device needs to be chosen in discussion with the patient, and its use taught and checked
Short-acting beta-agonist bronchodilators	The main therapy for treating the reversible component of airway obstruction which improves shortness of breath and increases exercise ability. Short-acting beta-agonists can be used as required for symptom relief. In more severe disease, they are best used regularly, every 2 to 4 hours, and can be taken in higher doses, perhaps in a nebulised format, to achieve a greater response
Anticholinergic drugs	Can be as efficacious as short-acting beta-agonists (and in some patients may provide greater symptom relief)
Beta-agonist and anticholinergic bronchodilators	May have an additive effect in improving exercise tolerance
Long-acting beta-agonist bronchodilators	Can improve exercise tolerance and quality of life in patients with COPD. Further studies on the role of this group of drugs in COPD are required
Theophyllines	Have a bronchodilator action but a fairly limited role in COPD, e.g. in patients who respond poorly to inhaled treatment or wake in the night with breathlessness

Table 6.5: Approaches to the management of COPD—continued

Inhaled corticosteroids	Have been shown to be effective in combination with long-acting bronchodilators in reducing the incidence of acute exacerbations of COPD
Other treatments	
Oral steroids	Have a role in acute exacerbations but ideally should not be used for long-term use
Antibiotics	Are of value for acute infective episodes of COPD, diagnosed in cases where there is increasing amounts of sputum, sputum purulence and increasing breathlessness. Courses of 7 days of antibiotics should be employed. There is no place for long-term antibiotics
Exercise	Should be encouraged regularly
Nutrition	Weight reduction may help breathlessness. Some patients with emphysema are underweight and may need advice on improved nutrition
Vaccination	Annual influenza vaccination is recommended. Pneumococcal vaccine is usually just given as one-off
Pulmonary rehabilitation	Has proven valuable in improving exercise tolerance and general well-being
Long term oxygen therapy (LTOT)	Patients with severe COPD and respiratory failure may benefit from LTOT. Specialist assessment, with blood gases, should be performed

staging of COPD should be according to the Gold Global Initiative in Obstructive Lung Disease.

TREATMENT OF COPD

A variety of guidelines are available to inform the management of COPD using drug and non-drug treatments. Table 6.5 summarises the variety of options.

Pulmonary embolism

A diagnosis of pulmonary embolism should be considered in any older person presenting with isolated dyspnoea and a raised respiratory rate, who develops symptoms suddenly after a period of prolonged immobilisation in hospital, on an aeroplane or in the home. Referral to hospital for chest X-ray, VQ scan or CT scan should be immediate if this diagnosis is suspected.

Reference

National Institute for Clinical Excellence (2003) Chronic Heart Failure — Management of chronic heart failure in adults in primary and secondary care. Clinical guideline 5, NICE, London.

Further reading

National Institute for Clinical Excellence (2004) Chronic obstructive pulmonary disease—National Clinical Guideline on management of chronic obstructive pulmonary disease in primary and secondary care THORAX MARCH 2004 (Volume 59 supplement).

CHAPTER 7

The older patient with change in bowel habits

CASE HISTORY

Mr. BH is an 85-year-old man with a past history of atrial fibrillation, heart failure and mild to moderate Alzheimer's disease. He was placed in a residential home two years earlier after he had fractured his femur. This was treated with hemiarthroplasty, and although he made a good recovery he did not feel confident enough to return home and made the decision to move into a private residential home.

At the time of his move he was taking digoxin 125 mcg/day, aspirin 75 mg/day and temazepam 10–20 mg at night when required. He settled quickly into the home's routine and had been well until a week ago when he developed intermittent diarrhoea. At the same time, the staff noticed that there was soiling of his sheets and his confusion had worsened. They call the GP who visits him after a morning surgery.

Having established the history as above, the GP examines Mr. BH. General examination reveals him to be disorientated in time and place. He knows his age and birth date but cannot recall the names of any of the staff. On MTS, he scores 5/10. Physical examination reveals he has a pulse of 76 per minute in atrial fibrillation with BP of 135/75 mmHg. He is apyrexial, well hydrated and there are no abnormal signs detected in the cardiovascular and respiratory systems. Examination of the abdomen reveals a palpable colon in the left iliac fossa, and on rectal examination he is noted to have hard faeces with normal anal tone. There are no neurological signs to suggest a CVA. Urine testing shows no blood, protein or leucocytes. The GP asks the staff to ensure that Mr. BH drinks plenty of fluids and prescribes glycerine suppositories for presumed faecal impaction. The GP says he would like to see how things go over the next few days and that the surgery should be called if Mr. BH's condition deteriorates. If there is no significant improvement over the next 48 hours, he will arrange for some blood samples with a possible view to referring for a geriatric opinion as to the cause of his confusion and change of bowel habit.

At the next weekly visit, the GP is asked to speak to Mr. BH's daughter who is extremely concerned about the recent deterioration in her father's condition. She says he has been losing weight and soiling his pants for the last two months and has asked her to take his clothes home for washing and not to inform the staff. On a few occasions, she has noted some blood on his underpants. She also states that while she wants to know if her father has a serious illness she does not wish her father to be 'pulled about', and certainly she would not wish him to have any operation.

Reassessment reveals that his confusion has improved with MTS 6/10. He still has a palpable colon in the abdomen but the rectum appears empty. On this occasion he admits he had loose stools a few weeks ago with occasional bleeding per rectum, and this stopped two weeks ago when he left out fruit and vegetables from his diet.

With the new facts, the GP decides that he may be dealing with more than faecal loading/impaction with overflow diarrhoea causing faecal soiling. He arranges for the district nurse to visit and take blood for a full blood count, urea and electrolytes, liver function tests, bone biochemistry and thyroid function tests. He contacts the secretary of Dr. HC, one of the local hospital consultants in geriatric medicine, and asks if she would call him back to discuss this patient's management.

Dr. HC phones back that day. They agree that with the recent change in bowel habits and rectal bleeding it is important to exclude colonic or high rectal tumour. But in view of the concerns expressed by the daughter, Dr. HC suggests that she sees the patient with his daughter within one week for an initial assessment and discussion.

Dr. HC meets Mr. BH in Outpatients the following week. Although Mr. BH does have some short-term memory difficulties, he is aware of his diarrhoea and rectal bleeding. He is embarrassed by the problem and realises it could be a sign of some serious underlying cause. When asked if he would be willing to undergo investigations in order to find the cause of his problem and decide the best treatment, he states that he has no objections. Dr. HC goes on to explain to Mr. BH and his daughter that many conditions can cause diarrhoea leading to faecal soiling and rectal bleeding, and it is important to confirm the cause by carrying out tests such as a sigmoidoscopy, X-ray examination following barium enema, or CT scan. Lastly, they are reassured that whatever the investigations show, no treatment will be given without their full consent.

Mr. BH is admitted to hospital for investigation. Sigmoidoscopy reveals no lesion up to 20 cm. Pneumocolon examination using CT scan reveals a polypoid mass in the sigmoid part of colon. Following this, biopsy is undertaken with the colonoscope. After confirming the presence of a well-differentiated adenocarcinoma, Dr. HC meets with the patient and his daughter to discuss the options for management. Agreement is reached to refer him to a colorectal surgeon for resection, which is carried out successfully. Postoperatively, Mr. BH develops delirium as a result of chest infection. However, twelve days after surgery he has made a good recovery and is discharged back to the home, mobile with a stick.

LEARNING POINTS FROM CASE HISTORY

- While the overwhelming majority of cases of faecal soiling in elderly patients are due to faecal loading/impaction other causes must always be considered.
- Rectal bleeding in association with change in bowel habit must be investigated fully.
- All investigations and treatment require consent from the patient.

Tutorial — change in bowel habits

Symptom of recent change in bowel habits (constipation and/or diarrhoea) should always raise suspicion of possible colorectal carcinoma. This is the second most common form of cancer in the UK, with over 90% of cases occurring in patients over the age of 50 years. In association with change in bowel habits, the older person may notice blood in the stools. Lesions affecting the proximal part of the colon and caecum may present insidiously with anaemia or late with signs and symptoms of secondary spread.

Risk factors for colon carcinoma include age over 50 years, presence of inflammatory bowel disease, polyposis syndrome and family history of breast or genital carcinoma in women.

Diagnosis may require examination of the rectum by sigmoidoscopy (which has a reported sensitivity of 48–50%) or colonoscopy (sensitivity of 80–90%), barium enema (sensitivity of 40%–60%) and pneumocolon examination using CT scanner. The latter is often a useful investigation in frail elderly who are not able to comply with the manoeuvres required by barium enema examination.

Part of the strategy for improving survival from colorectal carcinoma is early detection. In the USA, it is recommended that everyone over the age of 50 should have annual occult blood test and PR examination, with flexible sigmoidoscopy every 3–5 years. This is not a recommended practice in the UK. Only those with known risk factors, polyposis or ulcerative colitis are normally checked regularly.

Mortality in patients with colonic carcinoma is closely related to Duke's staging; while Dukes A carcinoma has mortality of 4% at 5 years, Dukes D carcinoma has a mortality of 19%.

Constipation

The range of normal bowel habit can vary from three stools a day to three stools per week. Individuals who complain of constipation may do so if their bowel movements have become less frequent than they used to be, or are finding it difficult to pass stools, having to strain. As a symptom, it is very common in immobilised older persons in whom gastrocolic reflex (peristalsis resulting from food entering the stomach) is impaired. In others, it may result from slow transit due to lack of colonic propulsion or may indicate an intrinsic colonic disease (e.g. carcinoma), or presence of a more general problem, such as hypothyroidism. Table 7.1 lists common causes that one should consider in an older person presenting with the symptom of constipation. If left untreated, severe constipation can lead to megacolon/megarectum which can not only lead to abdominal distension, but on occasion to sigmoid volvulus, particularly in institutionalised elderly.

ROME II CRITERIA FOR FUNCTIONAL CONSTIPATION

○ Straining at defaecation at least a quarter of the time.

○ Lumpy and hard stool at least a quarter of the time.

○ Sensation of incomplete evacuation at least a quarter of the time.

○ Two or more of the above should have been present for at least 12 weeks out of the preceding 12 months.

TREATMENT

The aim of treatment should be to produce stools of ideal consistency (i.e. not too hard or too soft) and bowel emptying to occur at a predictable time. General measures, such as exercise

Table 7.1: Causes of constipation	
General	• Idiopathic • Hypothyroidism • Hypercalcaemia • Uraemia • Depression
Large bowel	• Carcinoma • Irritable bowel syndrome
Drugs	• Analgesics, particularly those containing opiates
	• Antacids (containing aluminium or calcium) • Amiodarone • Anticholinergics (e.g. tricyclic antidepressants and antipsychotics) • Antidiarrhoeals • Antiparkinsonian drugs • Calcium-channel blockers • Calcium supplements • Clonidine • Disopyramide • Diuretics • Ferrous sulphate • Iron preparations • Laxatives (prolonged use) • Lithium • Nonsteroidal anti-inflammatory drugs • Opioids
Neurological	• Paraparesis • Dementia with or without frontal lobe damage

and a high-fibre diet, are useful in older people who are still active.

Little evidence is available as to the comparative effectiveness of bulk and non-bulking agents in the treatment of constipation (Table 7.2). Similarly, there is no good evidence that

Table 7.2: Laxatives

Type	Agent	Dose
Softening agents	Sodium docusate	100 mg tds
Stimulant laxatives	Senna Bisacodyl	3 tablets od 1 mg od
Osmotic	Macrogols (Movicol) Magnesium sulphate Lactulose	2 sachets bd 10 g od 30 ml bd
Bulking and stimulant	Manevac	4 g bd
Suppositories and enemas	Glycerol Micolette enemas	

laxatives prevent constipation. A stepped approach to laxative treatment would seem justified involving the use of the cheaper first before moving onto the more expensive ones.

Bulking agents, such as bran and ispaghula husk, work gently and are the most common type of laxatives (examples are Fybogel and Regulan). Studies have shown that they are better tolerated, with increased and better evacuation in comparison with sodium docusate, and are associated with a decrease in abdominal pain. Bulking agents should always be taken with plenty of fluids.

Stimulant laxatives work by increasing intestinal mobility by stimulating colonic nerves. Senna or bisacodyl have not been shown to be that effective, although there is some evidence that the combination of a bulk and a stimulant laxative (e.g. Manevac) can be more effective than lactulose. Osmotic laxatives (such as lactulose) work by increasing the amount of water in the stools. The senna and fibre combination may be more effective and cheaper than lactulose, but people who have limited mobility or are living in a residential/nursing home may require a stronger stimulant laxative, such as bisacodyl, or macrogols.

Macrogols (polyethylene glycols) are administered along with extra fluids, so they don't draw more water into the bowel from the body. Examples are Idrolax and Movicol. Macrogols may be of long-term benefit to patients with persistent constipation and faecal impaction. If laxatives are unsuccessful, Micolette enemas should be used in preference to phosphate enemas because side-effects have not been reported as much with their use. Those who have developed megacolon associated with chronic constipation benefit from fibre restriction and enemas once/twice per week. Detergents break down surface layers in the stool, letting water penetrate and soften it (e.g. docusate). It is recommended that danthron (expensive) should only be given for constipation in the terminally ill.

Diarrhoea

CAUSES

Apart from impaction of faeces and colonic carcinoma, diarrhoea can be produced by the following:

○ **Colonic diverticulosis.** Symptoms can vary from none to crampy abdominal pain (localised to the left iliac fossa and associated with diarrhoea or constipation) to diverticulitis and bleeding, requiring emergency admission for colonoscopy and/or surgery.

○ **Infections.** *Clostridium difficile* is a very important cause of diarrhoea in hospitals. It often follows antibiotic use. Although any antibiotic can lead to *Clostridium difficile* infection, the most commonly implicated antibiotics include cephalosporins, ampicillin, amoxicillin and clindamycin. The symptoms are caused by enterotoxin A, which leads to non-bloody diarrhoea, lower abdominal pain, low-grade fever and raised white cell count. In severe cases, it can lead to 'pseudomembranous colitis', producing dehydration, hypotension and toxic megacolon. Diagnosis can be made by immunoassay to detect toxin, cultures for *Clostridium difficile* and by sigmoidoscopy or colonoscopy where yellowish-grey pseudomembranes may be seen. Treatment consists of discontinuing the offending drug, general support including fluids, and oral metronidazole or vancomycin. Other infected causes of diarrhoea include *Shigella* colitis, *Escherichia coli* infection following consumption of contaminated meat and *Campylobacter jejuni* infections.

○ **Inflammatory bowel disease.** Chronic inflammatory bowel conditions, such as ulcerative colitis and Crohn's disease, may also affect older people. Symptoms and signs can be similar to those occurring in a younger person, although it is worth remembering that diarrhoea in older people may often lead to faecal incontinence.

○ **Colonic ischaemia.** In addition to bloody diarrhoea, an affected person may develop mild to moderate left lower abdominal pain, usually on the left side, with tenderness and pyrexia. Barium enema may reveal 'thumb printing' in the affected part. Treatment is conservative with antibiotics and fluids, unless gangrene develops.

○ **Steatorrhoea.** Malabsorption due to coeliac disease, bacterial overgrowth, chronic pancreatitis may not only develop diarrhoea but may have other features of malabsorption.

○ **Drugs.** Antibiotics, laxatives (abuse), cholestyramine.

○ **General.** Thyrotoxicosis, diabetes mellitus, hypoparathyroidism, carcinoid syndrome.

KEY LEARNING POINTS—CHANGE IN BOWEL HABIT

○ Constipation as a symptom is very common in immobilised older people.

○ General measures, such as exercise and high fibre diet, are useful in older people who complain of constipation and who are still active.

○ For laxative treatment of constipation, a stepped approach is recommended.

○ While there are many causes of diarrhoea, one should always consider and exclude two important and potentially treatable conditions: impaction of faeces and colonic carcinoma.

○ Change in bowel habits should always raise suspicion of possible colorectal carcinoma.

Further reading

Effectiveness of Laxatives in adults. Effective Health Care September 2001 Volume 7 Number 1.

Potter JM, Norton C, Cottenden A, eds. Bowel care in older people: research and practice. London: Royal College of Physicians; 2002.

CHAPTER 8

The older patient with continence problems

CASE HISTORY

On one of his regular visits to a local dually registered residential and nursing home, a GP is asked to review the following three patients.

Patient 1

Mrs. CPA, an 85-year-old woman with diverticular disease of the colon, has now developed diarrhoea and a tendency to soiling at night time. On one occasion, blood was noted on the sheet. Physical examination reveals no abnormal palpable masses, but rectal examination reveals blood on the examining finger, although no mass lesion is palpable. Further questioning reveals that Mrs. CPA has been known to have haemorrhoids, and these do intermittently bleed.

The GP suspects the diarrhoea and faecal incontinence may be related to a flare-up of diverticular disease, and the bleeding noted may be secondary to haemorrhoids. However, he cannot exclude bowel malignancy on clinical grounds. He discusses the situation with the patient who agrees to be referred for further investigation. He arranges for her to be seen at the local day hospital for proctoscopic/sigmoidoscopic examination.

Patient 2

Mr. CPB, a 92-year-old man with severe vascular dementia, has developed a tendency to smear his faeces on the wall. No other abnormal behaviour has been noted by the staff. Mr. CPB is not aware of his surroundings. He knows his Christian name but does not know his age or his date of birth. He appears a little agitated. As a result of this, physical examination is difficult but abdominal palpation reveals no obvious masses, and rectal examination reveals an empty rectum. Unable to obtain consent from the patient, the GP arranges to speak to his son on the telephone. They agree that it would be in Mr. CPB's best interest to investigate the problem further as there is potential to find a reversible cause for his continence problem. The GP takes blood for FBC, U&E, and LFTs and sends urine for culture and sensitivities. He feels it would be useful to discuss the case with the registrar in medicine for the elderly at the local hospital. The registrar agrees that the soiling of faeces may be related to behavioural problems associated with Alzheimer's dementia but also may suggest the presence of an acute illness worsening his confusion and altering his behaviour. The registrar arranges to see him in the day hospital within the next 48 hours. This assessment reveals no acute medical problems. The registrar arranges for a continence nurse specialist to visit Mr. CPB at the home and advise the staff on managing his faecal incontinence with appropriate aids and bowel retraining.

Patient 3

Mrs. CPC, aged 76, has just arrived at the home for a two-week respite admission while her family is away. She is severely disabled as a result of rheumatoid arthritis and requires a wheelchair for mobility. She is able to transfer from chair to commode, but because of difficulties in getting out of bed she uses pads for protection at night time. Over the last four days she has developed urgency with frequency of passing urine and as a result she has lost control of her bladder. On further tactful questioning, Mrs. CPC also admits to having had stress incontinence for several years. Examination of the abdomen is normal as is rectal examination. Pelvic examination reveals a dry atrophic vagina but no obvious prolapse. Urine testing with a dipstick reveals ++ of protein, ++ of blood and + for leucocytes. Based on these findings, the GP sends a sample of urine to the local microbiology laboratory for culture and sensitivities while starting her on trimethoprim 200 mg twice a day for three days. He arranges for the continence nurse specialist to assess Mrs. CPC while she is in the residential home.

LEARNING POINTS FROM CASE HISTORIES

- Urinary incontinence may result from simple conditions, such as urinary tract infection or atrophic vaginitis, which can be managed at home by the general practitioner.

- Faecal incontinence, like urinary incontinence, may result from common causes such as diarrhoea, and this again can be managed at home in most cases with treatment aimed at the underlying cause.

- Patients with severe dementia are not aware of what is socially acceptable and may develop faecal incontinence. In these individuals it may be advisable to use bowel retraining, once other treatable causes have been excluded.

- GPs, district nurses and residential home carers are in a good position to proactively address many risk factors for incontinence.

- Continence nurse specialists can contribute significantly to the assessment and management of any patient with continence problems.

- Patients may be reluctant to admit to continence problems.

Tutorial — incontinence of urine

Introduction

Incontinence of urine is one of the common treatable problems encountered in old age. Reported prevalence rates in the community for those over 65 years are 10–20% for females and approximately 10% for men. An even greater prevalence is noted in old people living in residential homes (25–30%) and in nursing homes (50%). The impact of incontinence on patients and carers can be most distressing and embarrassing, and often they are reluctant to discuss the problem with health professionals, thinking there is nothing that can be done.

Assessment of the patient with urinary incontinence

Incontinence is a symptom and not a pathological diagnosis, and an older person with urinary incontinence requires thorough clinical assessment, including accurate history and examination in order to define the problem and its possible causes. The history should explore the following areas:

○ exact nature and duration of symptoms
○ past medical history (including gynaecological and obstetric history in women)
○ current medication
○ impact on quality of life
○ environmental difficulties, e.g. location of toilet
○ diet and fluid intake.

Physical examination should include:

○ assessment of mobility

○ abdominal examination to detect masses, palpable bladder or loaded bowel

○ rectal examination to exclude faecal impaction and to detect prostatic size (in men)

○ pelvic examination in women

○ neurological examination, looking in particular at anal tone, perineal sensation and plantar responses

○ mental state examination

○ dipstick testing of urine for leucocytes and nitrites

○ post-void residual urine volume using a catheter or ultrasound where possible (normal is less than 100 ml)

In selected cases it may be necessary to proceed to specific tests such as urodynamics, measuring flow rates, urine volumes, bladder filling and pressures during voiding.

Causes

Urinary incontinence can develop not only as a result of conditions affecting the lower urinary tract, including the bladder, pelvic floor and the nervous system, but also from non-bladder causes such as problems with mobility leading to inability of an elderly person to get to the toilet in time, problems with transfers and presence of confusion.

Transient urinary incontinence may be caused by several conditions and these are best remembered by the mnemonics: DIAPPERS or DRIP (Box 8.1)

BOX 8.1: Mnemonics for remembering transient causes of urinary incontinence

DIAPERS

D Delirium

I   Infection—urinary tract or infection elsewhere, intercurrent illness

A Atrophic vaginitis/urethritis

P Pharmaceuticals (drugs)

P Psychological (depression)/lack of motivation

E Excessive urine production (hyperglycaemia, heart failure)

R Restricted/reduced mobility or poor access to toilet facilities

S Stool impaction

DRIP

D Delirium

R Restricted mobility

I   Infection, impaction, inflammation (atrophic vaginitis)

P Polyuria, pharmaceuticals

Management

The management of urinary incontinence is dependent upon the cause. The common conditions that can lead to urinary incontinence are discussed below. In all but the most transient cases, involvement of district nurses and continence nurse specialists should be considered. They have a vital role in patient/carer support and education, as well as expertise in the appropriate use of continence aids and appliances.

Urinary tract infection
When symptomatic, this requires appropriate antibiotic therapy, usually a three-day course. Choice of antibiotic may be determined by the sensitivity of the organism/bacteria producing the infection, but trimethoprim remains a reasonable first-choice empirical treatment for infections acquired in the community.

Atrophic vaginitis
Treatment consists of oestrogen cream applied locally or oestrogen tablets/capsules by mouth. Unopposed oestrogen therapy, even topical, should only be used as a short-term measure.

Drugs
Urinary incontinence may result as a side-effect of drugs, such as diuretics, sedatives, nonsteroidal anti-inflammatory drugs or calcium-channel blockers, and these individuals improve after cessation of the offending drug.

Constipation/faecal impaction
Depending on the degree/severity of impaction, which is best quantified by plain abdominal X-ray, this may require glycerine suppositories or enemas, as well as oral laxatives such as senna or sodium docusate.

Detrusor instability/detrusor overactivity
This is a term used for uninhibited bladder (detrusor) contractions and is responsible for 50–66% of incontinence in older people. The instability may be idiopathic or may be caused by obstruction, damage to the inhibitory centre or urinary tract infection. Symptoms include frequency, nocturia, urgency and urge incontinence.

Treatment. Bladder retraining works in some well-motivated individuals. In others, drugs can be tried, such as imipramine (also used as an antidepressant and has anticholinergic action), oxybutynin (antimuscarinic action) and tolterodine (fewer side-effects).

Stress incontinence

This is the second most common cause of incontinence in older females. It results from weakness of pelvic floor and bladder neck muscles in women. The damage to muscles usually occurs during childbirth or may result from oestrogen deficiency or uterine prolapse and cystocoele.

The diagnosis is made by examining the patient while standing, with the bladder full and asking her to cough. Procedures that have been shown to be effective in some older people include pelvic floor exercises (Kegel's) ± biofeedback, electrical therapy, tension-free vaginal tape procedure (recommended by National Institute for Clinical Excellence for women with uncomplicated urodynamic stress incontinence) and vaginal cones, which work better in 'young' elderly patients. In others, surgery to strengthen pelvic muscles may be useful. Although there are a number of procedures that can be performed surgically for stress incontinence, there is no agreement among the surgeons as to which is the best procedure. Recently, several devices have been developed to help patients with stress incontinence. The two forms of device are:

○ FemAssist, a device that covers the urethral orifice

○ Reliance, an intraurethral plug, which has to be removed each time the female wishes to pass urine.

Some patients with vaginal or uterine prolapse may benefit with ring or shelf pessaries.

Urinary retention with overflow

This results from unsustained detrusor activity in response to obstruction. This is the second most common cause of incontinence in men. Causes include prostatic hypertrophy, prostatic carcinoma, impaction of faeces, urethral stricture or mass lesion in the pelvis.

Prostatic hypertrophy. This can be treated by surgery, laser treatment or with drugs such as selective alpha-blockers (alfuzosin, doxazosin), which block sympathetic nervous activity and through this relax the smooth muscle component of prostatic obstruction, or finasteride which inhibits testosterone metabolism leading to reduction in prostate size.

Prostatic carcinoma. Although this may present with urinary retention with overflow, it can be asymptomatic, cause local pain or present with symptoms of secondary spread to bone. Diagnosis is suggested by an irregular enlarged prostate on rectal examination, associated with raised prostate specific antigen (PSA). However, in relation to PSA, it is worth remembering that the level can increase with age, with increase in prostatic size and with prostatitis. Therefore, interpretation of raised values needs to be considered carefully. Early localised disease may not require any intervention, while those with symptoms require surgery, radiotherapy or hormonal therapy (flutamide, goserelin or cyproterone) for those with secondary spread to bone.

Neurogenic bladder

This results from damage to neural control of the bladder. Depending upon the lesion, different types of incontinence may result. These include:

○ **Uninhibited bladder.** This may be found in patients with stroke, Parkinson's disease, multi-infarct dementia or frontal lobe tumour. Loss of voluntary cerebral inhibition leads to detrusor hyperreflexia, resulting in symptoms of frequency, urgency and urge incontinence.

○ **Reflex bladder.** This often results after injury to the spinal cord. The patient with reflex bladder has bladder detrusor hyper-reflexia without sensation; therefore the bladder empties when it fills to a certain volume and leads to incomplete emptying. The person is not aware of the incontinence.

○ **Atonic bladder.** Causes include diabetes mellitus, trauma from pelvic surgery and tabes dorsalis. Symptomatically, these patients have retention of urine with overflow (dribbling), with or without sensation. The typical symptoms are a recurrent urinary tract infection, associated with high residual urine. The main finding is detrusor areflexia, with variable loss of sensation depending upon the site of the lesion.

Normal pressure hydrocephalus
Classically, persons with normal pressure hydrocephalus present with a triad of progressive gait disorder, cognitive impairment and urinary incontinence. If detected early and treated with a shunt or repeated lumbar punctures, symptoms can be improved.

Delirium/dementia
A confused or demented person may not appreciate when and where to empty the bladder appropriately.

Non-urinary tract causes leading to 'functional incontinence'
The important factors include the 'five Ms': motivation, medical illness, mobility, mental state and manual dexterity. Clearly, management relates to addressing the underlying cause.

OTHER TREATMENTS

Patients who are undergoing or who fail to respond to treatment for incontinence may require:

○ **Incontinence pads and sheets.** These can be disposable or washable, and vary in their absorbent properties and size.

○ **External devices.** Condom catheters/penile sheaths may be useful for male patients. These can be self-adhesive or supplied with separate adhesive strips, but unfortunately they still have the tendency to fall off easily or can be pulled off by confused persons.

○ **Indwelling catheters.** For short-term use, a catheter made of latex is preferred, but those requiring catheterisation on a long-term basis should have a silicone-coated catheter. Individuals in whom a catheter is placed temporarily should have the catheter clamped for two hours daily to retain bladder capacity. It is worth noting that catheterisation is not without risk. Complications include infection, encrustation leading to catheter blockage and bladder spasm. A catheter specimen of urine (CSU) may produce mixed growth or significant growth of organisms on culture, but patients only require treatment with antibiotics if they have associated symptoms.

Tutorial — faecal incontinence

Faecal incontinence (defined as involuntary or inappropriate passage of faeces) is one of the most distressing symptoms to cope with for patients and carers. It is said to occur in approximately 3% of elderly people living at home and in up to 20–45% of elderly people in continuing care beds. While age-associated changes, such as diminution in anal squeeze pressure or decrease in the distension of the rectum (which produces the desire to void), may predispose to faecal incontinence, there are specific conditions that lead to faecal incontinence. The common causes include:

○ Immobility—this can lead to difficulties getting to the toilet on time and loss of gastrocolic reflex.

○ Difficulty in dressing/undressing (removing clothes).

○ Factors relating to access to toilet.

○ Constipation/faecal impaction with overflow. The presence of hard faeces causes the mucosa to secrete mucus which results in soiling by liquid or semi-solid faeces several times a day. It also causes impaired rectal sensation and anorectal reflex, with reduction in resting anal pressure.

○ Diarrhoea from any cause, e.g. infection, drugs (including laxative abuse), irritable bowel syndrome.

○ Anal sphincter weakness with associated fall in squeeze pressure.

○ Rectal prolapse.

○ Carcinoma of rectum.

○ Diverticular disease of colon.

○ Inflammatory bowel disease, e.g. ulcerative colitis or Crohn's disease.

○ Dementia ('uninhibited incontinence'). Patients become incontinent because they cannot appreciate when and where to void, or because they cannot resist faeces entering the rectum following a mass peristalsis, which may result in the stimulation of the gastrocolic reflex resulting from food entering the stomach.

○ Delirium.

○ Other neurological conditions, including multiple strokes, diabetic autonomic neuropathy, multiple sclerosis and pudendal nerve damage.

Management

Management of elderly people with faecal incontinence includes identifying the cause(s) and their treatment. In the majority of cases, faecal incontinence is treatable and/or preventable.

In relation to anorectal weakness incontinence, young persons do relatively well with sphincter and pelvic muscle exercises and surgery, and older persons can be helped by maintaining a firm stool.

Patients with dementia can be best helped by prompted or scheduled toileting, or a regimen of planned defecation with use of an enema or suppositories 1–3 times per week, with intermittent use of constipating agents to prevent leakage between enemas.

A small minority with intractable faecal incontinence will require appropriate protective clothing. Recently, faecal collection bags (which can be placed around the anus using an adhesive tape) have been introduced. These are particularly useful for elderly patients who are immobile or have severe diarrhoea. The other important aspect of faecal as well as urinary incontinence is odour control. Many deodorants are available to achieve this.

KEY LEARNING POINTS — CONTINENCE PROBLEMS

○ Incontinence of urine is one of the common treatable problems encountered in old age.

○ Incontinence is a symptom and not a pathological diagnosis, and an older person with urinary incontinence requires thorough clinical assessment, including accurate history and examination.

○ Only in a few selected cases will it be necessary to proceed to specific tests, such as urodynamics measuring flow rates, urine volumes, bladder filling and pressures during voiding.

○ Management of urinary incontinence is dependent upon the cause, and simple causes such as urinary tract infection or atrophic vaginitis can be managed at home by the general practitioner.

○ Faecal incontinence is common and is said to occur in approximately 3% of elderly people living at home and in up to 20%–45% of elderly in continuing care beds.

○ In the majority of cases, faecal incontinence is treatable and/or preventable, treatment being aimed at the cause.

Further reading

National Institute for Clinical Excellence. Guidance on the use of tension-free vaginal tape (Gynecare TVT) for stress incontinence. London: National Institute for Clinical Excellence; 2003.

Potter JM, Norton C, Cottenden A, eds. Bowel care in older people: research and practice. London: The Royal College of Physicians; 2002.

Report of the Royal College of Physicians. Incontinence — causes, management and provision of services. London: The Royal College of Physicians; 1995.

CHAPTER 9

The older patient with skin problems

CASE HISTORY

Mrs. SK is an 84-year-old widow who lives alone and is normally very healthy and independent. Recently, she has been complaining bitterly of dry, itching skin. She also has had a 'pimple' on her nose for several months which won't go away. She is on no regular medication and her weight is steady.

The general practitioner

The GP takes a detailed history of her complaints. Apart from the skin problems, she is well. She examines Mrs. SK and finds her skin is generally dry, and there are some excoriations on her arms and legs due to scratching. She has some small bruises and a variety of moles, keratoses and skin tags on her trunk, but none of these look worrying. However, the spot on her nose does have a slightly irregular edge which makes the GP think of a possible basal cell carcinoma. She is not jaundiced or uraemic, and there are no abdominal swellings. She has a regular pulse, normal blood pressure and moderately swollen ankles with slightly varicose leg veins. The GP arranges blood tests (full blood count, urea and electrolytes, random glucose and liver function test) and prescribes another emollient and an antihistamine which is supposed to be non-sedating. She asks Mrs. SK to return in two weeks to discuss the results, see if the itching has improved and to review the lesion on her nose.

When Mrs. SK and the GP meet two weeks later the blood tests results are back and are all within normal limits. Mrs. SK is still very itchy. The antihistamines did cause sedation, and in fact one night after she had taken one she had had a fall and cut her right lower leg when she got up to go to the toilet. The lesion on her nose has not changed.

At this point, the GP feels the need for specialist advice. She considers a dermatological referral but decides that a more general assessment at the local geriatric day hospital would be more appropriate given Mrs. SK's age and the nature of her problems. Mrs. SK agrees to this and the GP writes a referral letter outlining the history and the findings on examination and investigation.

The hospital consultant

The hospital consultant sees Mrs. SK at the day hospital and spends some time going through the history and examination. He does not suspect any underlying systemic condition causing her skin dryness. He is confident that the minor bruising on her hands and arms does not represent any clotting problem or suggest abuse but is due to senile purpura. He does feel that the lesion on her nose is likely to be a basal cell carcinoma (BCC) and will need treatment. He also finds that she is developing a venous ulcer on her right lower leg which will need compression dressings. He examines the various other skin lesions about which Mrs. SK is concerned. He identifies some senile keratoses and Campbell de Morgan spots and reassures her that these are common changes seen in ageing skin and not a cause for alarm.

The consultant gathers that Mrs. SK has been bathing twice a day to try and moisturise her skin, and that it is actually rather difficult for her to apply the emollient cream which she has been prescribed as she can't reach all over her body. He explains to her that this may actually be making her skin more dry and advises that she bathes no more than alternate days and uses a moisturising cream as a cleanser instead of her regular soap. He writes back to the GP explaining his findings and saying that he has referred Mrs. SK to a dermatologist colleague for surgical removal of the BCC. He suggests that the district nurse should be asked to visit Mrs. SK to apply emollients to her dry skin and compression dressings to her leg ulcer.

Tutorial — skin problems

The changes which we associate with ageing skin take place slowly over many years and are the result of the combined effects of genetic factors, disease and environmental exposure (e.g. wind, sun and smoking). It is now recognised that the changes due to chronic ultraviolet radiation (photoaging or dermatoheliosis) are distinct from and more severe than those resulting from intrinsic or true ageing of skin. Anatomical changes in the ageing skin result in altered physiological activity and eventually increased susceptibility to disease. In old age there is decreased epidermal renewal and tissue repair. Hair and nail growth declines as does the secretion from eccrine, apocrine and sebaceous glands. The dermis becomes thinner, less dense and less elastic. Cutaneous vascular supply is reduced and there is a decrease in number and size of mast cells and fibroblasts. These processes result in skin which is dryer, rougher, more wrinkled and lax. There is also an increased incidence of generally benign lesions, such as solar keratoses and telangiectasia.

Presentation of skin complaints

Dryness, often associated with itching, is the most common dermatological complaint in the elderly. Rough, dry scaling skin, sometimes known as xerosis, affects at least 75% of people over 64 years old. It is more common in women than men and tends to be worse at night and in winter. Xerosis is due in part to decreased eccrine sweating, decreased sebum production, decreased water content of the stratum corneum and decreased cohesion of corneocytes. It is cosmetically undesirable, uncomfortable, itchy and can be a basis for eczematous eruptions and infection. Some elderly people will respond to dry skin by frequent bathing, but without the use of emollients this can dry the skin further. Scratching itchy dry skin can lead to eczematous change and eventually infection. The generalised dryness which occurs in xerosis should help to differentiate this from seborrhoeic dermatitis, which is also common in older people and occurs characteristically on the chest, face, scalp and ears. Asteatotic eczema or eczema craquelatum (or craquelé) is a transient form of dermatitis often seen in the elderly and related to low humidity and frequent bathing. Asteatotic eczema occurs usually on extensor limb surfaces and trunk. The skin takes the appearance of 'crazy paving' and is itchy and often tender.

Apart from dry skin conditions, other common skin problems which elderly patients may present can be broadly classified into four groups: malignant/premalignant, infective, vascular and autoimmune (Table 9.1)

Assessment of the elderly skin

As at any age, the key to diagnosis and treatment is based on thorough and logical history and examination. Key areas in the history (Box 9.1) would be to seek the nature and duration of symptoms, presence of itching, affected body sites, general medical history, drug, occupational, family, recreational and travel history. In the elderly, a systematic review to discover any other current symptoms is important to exclude underlying and undiagnosed systemic illness. It is also important to make an assessment of the patient's function at home and to seek the patient and/or carer's views on the cause of any skin problem. Ideally, all patients should be examined undressed and in good light. Examining only exposed parts may miss clues given by distribution of lesions.

Table 9.1: Simple classification of skin problems in the elderly

Dry skin conditions	Xerosis Seborrhoeic dermatitis Asteatotic eczema
Malignant/premalignant conditions	Senile keratoses Basal cell carcinoma Squamous cell carcioma Bowen's disease Malignant melanoma
Infective conditions	Scabies Intertrigo Cellulitis Flea bites
Vascular conditions	Telangiectases Thrombophlebitis Senile purpura Erythema ab igne Pressure sores Leg ulcers
Autoimmune conditions	Pemphigoid Lichen sclerosus

BOX 9.1: Key areas to cover in history of elderly patients with skin problems

- Nature and duration of symptoms
- Presence of itch
- Affected body sites
- General medical history
- Drug history
- Occupational history
- Family history
- Recreational history
- Travel history
- Patient's/carer's views on cause

Investigation is not always necessary in the management of skin problems, which can often be diagnosed on the basis of history and examination. In suspected fungal infections, mycological examination is indicated on scrapings from skin lesions. There is a limited role for patch testing if allergic contact dermatitis is suspected. For cutaneous lesions which are atypical or where malignancy is suspected, a dermatological opinion should be sought and diagnostic biopsy will usually be necessary. Generalised pruritus in the elderly should be investigated initially with full blood count, chest X-ray, serum urea and electrolytes, glucose, liver and thyroid function tests and an autoantibody screen. These tests are justified in order to exclude the commoner systemic associations of generalised itching as shown in Box 9.2. More specialised subsequent investigation will depend on the history and results of initial screening tests. Generalised pruritus should also alert to the possibility of primary skin disorders, such as scabies and pemphigoid which are also more common in older people.

BOX 9.2: Commoner diseases associated with generalised itching

- Diabetes mellitus
- Hyperthyroidism
- Hypothyroidism
- Liver disease
- Primary biliary cirrhosis
- Chronic renal failure
- Polycythaemia
- Haemochromatosis
- Lymphoma
- Parasitosis
- Drug ingestion

Treatment of dry skin in the elderly

If no systemic cause is suspected or discovered then dry skin should be vigorously treated with emollients such as aqueous cream or E45 cream. Whilst the importance of hygiene should be stressed in treating elderly people with dry or itchy skin, it is also important to advise them not to use soap on their skin. Most ordinary soaps significantly reduce the hydrophilic property of the stratum corneum, which tends to aggravate dryness. Soap can be substituted with aqueous cream, emulsifying ointment, Unguentum M or some proprietary synthetic skin detergents often combined with moisturiser. Emollient treatment should be accompanied by avoidance of known skin irritants and general advice on fluids and nutrition. Humidifiers in central heating systems may be helpful, and patients should be advised not to scrub the skin or use the towel too vigorously after the bath or shower. Topical steroid creams should be avoided in the treatment of dry skin in the elderly, as the skin is already thin and fragile and may become more so with their prolonged use (Box 9.3).

BOX 9.3: Summary of management of dry skin in the elderly

- Exclude external irritants
- Exclude systemic illness
- Attention to adequate fluids and nutrition
- Skin hygiene
- Vigorous use of emollients
- Replace soap with substitute
- Avoid skin scrubbing
- Humidifier

The reason that itching is often associated with dry skin in the elderly remains unclear. Hypotheses include frequent penetration of irritants through an abnormal stratum corneum and an altered sensory threshold due to mild neuropathy. Patients can be reassured that itching should decrease as skin moisture improves with emollient therapy. Systemic antihistamines may give relief of itching but should be used with caution in the elderly as they can cause drowsiness and sometimes confusion and falls.

Skin conditions in the elderly

PRE-MALIGNANT AND MALIGNANT SKIN CONDITIONS

Senile keratoses

Sometimes known as solar or actinic keratoses these are scaly, hyperpigmented lesions which develop on exposed areas of skin. They look like dry, cracked plaques. They have a very low malignant potential but can over time progress to squamous cell carcinoma. They can be treated with cryotherapy, 5-fluouracil cream or local excision if large.

Basal cell carcinoma

Also known as rodent ulcers because of their tendency to local destruction, these are commonly related to sun exposure and usually occur on the face above a line joining the chin to the ear lobe. They have raised irregular edges, may be ulcerated and often have a pearly border. They should be referred early for excision, radiotherapy or cryotherapy.

Squamous cell carcinoma (SCC)

These usually arise on sun-damaged skin but are also seen in scars, longstanding gravitational ulcers or on the lips of smokers. SCC usually presents as a hyperkeratotic, ulcerated, rapidly expanding nodule. Local destruction may be extensive and metastatic spread to local draining lymph nodes and beyond will occur if not treated promptly. Surgical excision is the usual treatment.

Bowen's disease

This is a form of intraepidermal carcinoma in situ which can rarely progress to squamous cell carcinoma. It presents as an isolated scaly, pink plaque, rather like a patch of psoriasis and usually on the trunk. If untreated, the lesions slowly expand over a period of years and a very small proportion develop into metastasizing SCC. Surgical excision is recommended. There is difference of opinion as to whether patients with Bowen's disease have a higher than expected incidence of unrelated internal malignancy.

Malignant melanoma

This is a malignant tumour of epidermal melanocytes. Incidence is increasing in all parts of the world. They are twice as common in women as men. They commonly present as an irregularly pigmented macule or plaque with irregular margins. Elderly patients may have large numbers of pigmented lesions and it can be difficult to identify suspicious features. The main indications of possible malignancy are change in size or irregularity in shape or colour. There are four main histopathological types of melanoma (superficial spreading melanoma, lentigo maligna melanoma, nodular melanoma and acral lentiginous melanoma). Lentigo maligna melanoma occurs particularly on the exposed skin of the elderly, usually the face. An irregularly pigmented and shaped macule (lentigo maligna) may have been enlarging slowly for many years as an in situ melanoma before an invasive nodule (lentigo maligna melanoma) appears.

Melanomas are fast growing and it is essential that an early diagnosis is made. The only effective treatment is excision.

INFECTIVE SKIN CONDITIONS

Scabies

Scabies is a persistent itchy skin eruption caused by cutaneous infestation with the mite *Sarcoptes scabei*. It is related to poor housing and hygiene conditions. Patients complain of severe and persistent itch worse at night. Typical sites are the finger webs, sides of fingers, wrists, axillae, umbilicus and groin. Examination may reveal excoriated papules with linear burrows extending from them. In longstanding cases, secondary infection with pustules and crusting may be seen. Firm diagnosis can be made by extracting the mite from a burrow for microscopic examination. Treatment should be given to all the household. An effective scabicide (e.g. malathion 0.5% liquid) should be applied to the whole body from the neck down after bathing. This should be left on the skin for 24 hours and then washed off in a hot bath. All clothing and bed linen should be washed. Itching may continue for a few days after treatment. It is wise to provide written instructions on treatment if possible.

Intertrigo

This describes a fungal dermatitis occurring in skin flexures, typically axilla, groin or under the breast. The cause is the yeast *Candida albicans*. Lesions are shiny, confluent and red, often with satellite lesions and occasionally pustules around them. Diagnosis is clinical but should be confirmed by examining swabs for organisms. Risk factors for fungal infection should always be considered (i.e. recent antibiotics, diabetes or immune suppression). Treatment involves keeping the affected skin surfaces apart and dry and applying an antifungal agent such as clotrimazole solution or cream. Topical steroids should be avoided as they promote the further growth of *Candida*.

Cellulitis

Cellulitis is a cutaneous infection usually due to streptococcus. It presents as a raised hot tender erythematous area of skin. Often there has been a break in the skin or leg ulcer in the affected area. Fever and lymphadenopathy are common. Swabs should be taken and treatment commenced with systemic antibiotics. In general, penicillin V is the first line of treatment for cellulitis, but in the elderly there is more often a variety of organisms involved and a broader spectrum of flucloxacillin alone or in combination with penicillin may be preferred.

Flea bites

Flea bites may present in pet owners as multiple itchy papules around ankles and calves. Management mainly involves disinfesting the pets, furniture and carpets for which the advice of a vet and/or environmental health department should be sought. Hydrocortisone ointment or calamine lotion will relieve itching until the bites resolve.

VASCULAR SKIN CONDITIONS

Telangiectases

These are permanently dilated and visible small vessels in the skin. Whilst they can be associated with various pathologies, including hereditary, neurological, hepatic (spider naevi) and connective tissue disorders, they are commonly seen in the exposed skin of the elderly and need not generally cause concern.

Thrombophlebitis

This is thrombosis in an inflamed vein. If the affected vein is varicose, it will be red and feel like a tender cord. The leg may be generally inflamed, making a distinction from cellulitis difficult. Migratory superficial thrombophlebitis can be associated with underlying malignancy. Treatment for thrombophlebitis consists of rest and nonsteroidal anti-inflammatory drugs. Antibiotics rarely help.

Senile purpura

Senile purpura is a term sometimes used to describe the easy bruising often seen in elderly people. It is more common on the hands and arms, and presumed to be due to easy rupture of small vessels resulting from reduced collagen elasticity and vessel tethering. However, bruising in the elderly should not be easily dismissed as it can be an important manifestation of systemic disease or elder abuse.

Erythema ab igne

This term describes the appearance of skin, usually on the legs, which has been exposed to long-term local heat (e.g. from an electric fire or hot water bottle). The erythema is usually reticulate, reflecting the underlying vascular network and may have some scaling.

Leg ulcers

Leg ulcers are common and difficult to treat. Estimates are that one in fifty people over 80 have active leg ulcers. Resultant pain and immobility can often lead to isolation and depression. Approximately 50% of leg ulcers are due to venous stasis, 10% to arterial disease and 30–40% are mixed. The first sign of venous ulceration is often a patch of superficial inflammation which may be itchy. The surface then breaks down to form the ulcer. This often becomes chronic, with 40% persisting after one year and 10% presenting for over five years. Initial assessment of any patient with leg ulcer should include full history and examination to exclude unusual causes, such as skin malignancy or arteritis. Presence of infection should also be considered. Pulses should be examined and mobility assessed. The ulcer should be accurately described and measured.

Ulcers can usually be managed at home with the help of district nursing colleagues (Sarkar & Ballantyne 2000). In most primary care teams, the nurses will be the experts in ulcer management. They will check that the ulcer is clean and select appropriate dressings and change intervals to ensure this. They will apply compression bandages and stockings, which are the mainstay of venous ulcer treatment. However, it is important to remember that an arterial component to an ulcer is common in the elderly, and the inappropriate use of compression bandaging on an arterial ulcer can be disastrous. For this reason, the assessment of arterial circulation using Doppler studies is desirable before compression treatment commences. Compression reduces oedema and aids venous return. The bandages are applied over the ulcer dressing, from the forefoot to just below the knee, and left on for two to seven days at a time. General measures such as weight reduction, elevation of the affected limb and walking are all helpful. The GP is likely to be involved by the nurse if oedema is difficult to reduce, if infection is found or if pain is not controlled by simple analgesia. An ulcer will not heal if the leg is swollen and the patient chair-bound. Whilst it may be tempting to treat oedema with diuretics, they are only likely to help if the swelling is due to cardiac failure. For oedema due to hypostasis, elevation and pressure bandaging are the correct approach.

If infection is suspected, a swab should be taken. However, antibiotics should only be used if surrounding cellulitis is present, in which case a broad-spectrum agent such as flucloxacillin can be useful. If anaerobes are suspected due to the characteristic odour, metronidazole may be substituted or added.

The involvement of a physiotherapist for leg exercises, elevation, massage and ultrasound treatment to the skin around the ulcer can also be very helpful in management. Sometimes, a few days bedrest may help. Admission to hospital for elevation and intensive physical treatment is sometimes needed for severe ulcers, but patients in these circumstances may stay in hospital for several weeks and the ulcers often break down again when they go home. Surgery with autologous pinch or split-thickness grafts has an occasional place for intractable ulcers.

It is important to remember that although good evidence is now available on the most effective treatments for leg ulcers, these measures may not always be acceptable to elderly patients. Therefore, compliance is an issue. Pressure bandages and leg elevation, for example, may be uncomfortable for many people. Compromise and negotiation are part of the skills required in managing the problem.

Pressure sores

Necrosis of skin, fat and muscle caused by pressure often combined with shearing force and/or friction can occur rapidly in elderly people. Typical sites include skin overlying the sacrum, greater trochanter, ischial tuberosity and heels. Risk factors include acute and chronic illness, immobility, incontinence, poor nutrition, reduced sensation, neurological disease, recent surgery and terminal illness. Drugs such as sedatives or analgesics can also increase risk. Approximately 80% of pressure sores are superficial and 20% are deep. Sores begin as a local area of redness which progresses to a superficial blister or erosion. If pressure continues, deeper damage occurs often with the development of a black plug which covers a deep ulcer. Prevention is the most important aspect of management. Attention must be given to the general condition of the patient, treating any underlying medical problems and/or nutritional deficiencies. All immobile patients should be turned regularly and provided, wherever possible, with anti-pressure mattresses (NICE 2003). Debridement of sores, regular cleansing and absorbent dressings are important. Infection is common, and in-hospital pseudomonas and MRSA pose particular threats. Antibiotics are generally only used if infection is spreading. The

NHS National Institute of Clinical Excellence (NICE 2001) has published clinical guidelines on 'Pressure ulcer risk assessment and prevention'. Again nurses are the experts in care of pressure areas.

AUTOIMMUNE SKIN CONDITIONS

Pemphigoid
Pemphigoid is an autoimmune bullous disease. It presents as a chronic, sometimes itchy, blistering illness in elderly patients. Multiple tense bullae may be seen, often in flexural areas. Although pemphigoid is described as self-limiting, if untreated it can cause much discomfort and fluid loss from ruptured bullae. Steroids and immune suppressants are therefore used with caution. Doses are gradually reduced to a maintenance level which may need to continue for one or two years.

Lichen sclerosus
This is a chronic inflammatory skin disorder which mainly affects the vulval and perianal area in older women but can affect penis and anal area in men. Diagnosis requires biopsy. Steroids are the mainstay of treatment and use in a small increased risk of squamous cell carcinoma.

KEY LEARNING POINTS— SKIN PROBLEMS

○ A wide variety of skin problems can affect older people, and some can significantly affect quality of life.

○ Most problems can be identified by thorough history and examination.

○ Dryness, often associated with itching, is the most common dermatological complaint in the elderly.

o It is important when assessing any skin complaint in older people to be alert to the possibility of dermatological malignancy or underlying systemic disease.

o Always be aware of the risk of venous ulceration after injury to the lower legs in the elderly.

o Awareness of risk factors is essential in the prevention of pressure sores in elderly patients.

o Most skin problems in the elderly can be adequately managed in general practice.

References

National Institute for Clinical Excellence. Pressure ulcer risk assessment and prevention: inherited clinical guideline B. London: National Institute for Clinical Excellence; 2001.

National Institute for Clinical Excellence. Pressure ulcer prevention: pressure ulcer risk assessment and prevention, including the use of pressure-relieving devices (beds, mattresses and overlays) for the prevention of pressure ulcers in primary and secondary care (Clinical guideline 7). London: National Institute for Clinical Excellence; 2003.

Sarkar PK, Ballantyne S. Management of leg ulcers. Postgrad Med J 2000; 76(901):674–682.

Further reading

Champion RH, et al. Textbook of Dermatology. 6th edn. Oxford: Blackwell; 1998.

Pathy MSJ, ed. Principles and Practice of Geriatric Medicine. 3rd edn. Chichester: Wiley; 1998.

CHAPTER **10**

The older patient
with vision or
hearing problems

CASE HISTORY 1

Mr. V, aged 82, comes to see the practice nurse for the removal of sutures from the small lacerations on his forehead that he received in a road traffic accident a week ago. He was driving carefully on his usual route home from the shops in the evening when he turned right and collided with an oncoming vehicle. 'I just did not see it coming', he said. Fortunately the impact speed was low, and he only sustained a few cuts around the forehead, which were sutured in the local A&E department, but his car was badly damaged.

Tutorial — visual loss

Visual loss is an uncommon complaint in general practice, except when an acute red eye or the more ominous symptoms of retinal detachment bring someone urgently to the surgery. More often it appears because something else (a fall or a road traffic accident) reveals it. Yet visual impairment is common amongst older people, and the prevalence increases with advancing age. In community-based surveys of older people undertaken in the United Kingdom, visual acuity of less than 6/12 has been found in around 2% of subjects aged 65 to 74, and around 20% of subjects aged 75 and over (Wormald et al 1992). This level of visual acuity is below the UK driving requirements, and it is possible that Mr. V's accident was due to poor acuity made worse by twilight. The crash rate per driver amongst those aged 65 and over is low, probably because older drivers tend to drive shorter distances and avoid driving at night, in heavy traffic or in bad weather. However, the crash rate per mile driven for older drivers is higher than that for younger adults, and is lower than only one other group, teenagers. The increase in the pace and density of modern traffic puts older drivers at a disadvantage, although this may diminish as a generation who learned to drive late in life gives way to one which grew up in an automotive society. Right-of-way and turning accidents occur particularly frequently with older drivers (Waller 1991), and may be due to age-related changes in vision that cause problems with:

○ merging traffic streams

○ vehicles appearing unexpectedly in their peripheral vision

○ judging own speed and that of approaching vehicles

○ reading poorly-lit road signs or dim vehicle information displays.

Prevalence

Population studies in the UK suggests that 14% of the population aged 65 and over (van der Pols et al 2000) and 12% of the 75 and over age group are visually impaired, the prevalence rising rapidly with advancing age, especially for women. A general practitioner with a list size of 1800 in a demographically average area will have about 250 patients aged 65 and over, of whom 35 will have significant visual impairment, even when wearing glasses. Assuming that the rule of halves applies, some 17 of these people will have visual impairment that is unknown to others, and which they have not disclosed or even admitted to themselves for reasons that we will discuss later. Cataract and age-related macular degeneration (AMD) are the commonest causes of this visual loss, producing 63% and 20% of loss respectively in people aged 65 and over in a UK community survey. Refraction defects are also very common and are uncorrected or inadequately corrected in a quarter of those aged 65 and over and in almost half of those aged 75 and over (Smeeth 1998). Macular degeneration, with its bilateral clouding of central vision, is a particularly disabling impairment, affecting nearly one in five of those aged 85 or more. Glaucoma is the leading cause of acquired blindness, but is also relatively uncommon (occurring in 7% of people in the same survey) and now routinely screened for by opticians.

Despite the easy availability of free eye tests in the high street and a culture that does not stigmatise visual impairment in the way it does deafness, community surveys of older populations suggest that over half the visual impairment in this age group could potentially be reduced with treatment, particularly cataract surgery or refractive correction (Wormald et al 1992). General practice is inevitably one setting where assessment of vision and timely intervention can take place, and it may be the most important as GPs are likely to see the older people who have not visited the optician recently. Before discussing how best to identify this group, we do need some sense of what their poor vision really means to their health.

Impact

Visual impairment is associated with a substantial diminution in quality of life comparable with that produced by diabetes and stroke (Brown et al 2003). Interestingly, diabetes has its own national service framework, and stroke is an important element in the NSF for older people. However, visual impairment has a lower profile. Visual loss undermines independence in performing the tasks of everyday daily living, interferes with social activities, is associated with depression, falls and hip fracture, and with higher all-cause mortality in women if not in men. Sudden or severe loss of vision can be an overwhelming personal and family catastrophe, affecting the patient's mobility, work and personal relationships, yet if the change in eyesight is slow (which is the experience of most older people with impaired vision) it is easier for others to underestimate the extent of its impact.

Findings from a recent UK study of 1683 individuals aged 55 and over (Frost et al 2001) suggest a substantial national prevalence of vision-related quality of life (VR-QOL) impairment, and are consistent with earlier studies linking ocular disease with advancing age and social deprivation. The authors argue that consideration should be given to directing resources more carefully towards groups at higher risk of VR-QOL impairment, in particular the very elderly and socially deprived. There is a clue here for general practitioners, who might opt to focus attention on their oldest patients.

Visual problems in older people may go unreported and unrecognised for a number of reasons, including:

○ Decreased patient expectation in later life, and the attribution of changes to 'old age'.
○ A belief that nothing can be done to help, and the normalisation of the changes that are being experienced.
○ Failure by the patient to recognise their visual loss, especially if it is slowly progressive and they (or others) can compensate for it. Stopping a hobby that involves close work may be accepted as inevitable, and when it gets difficult to see the products on the supermarket shelf someone else may take over the shopping.
○ The presence of another problem, which dominates the perception of difficulties. Mr. V may be a good example of this, for his injuries need attention and his car needs repair.
○ Fears about treatment such as cataract surgery, although surgical risks are low, postoperative discomfort limited and the gain in vision almost always significant (assuming no retinal pathology) and sometimes dramatic.
○ The perceived or real costs of testing or treatment, particularly the purchase of new glasses.
○ The stigma (and fear) of blindness.

We should not forget that sensory defects disable all who come into contact with them, including doctors and nurses, whose ability to communicate sensitively and empathically with a visually impaired patient may diminish. Professionals may give up trying to communicate, avoid or minimise contact, and inadvertently indicate that the partially sighted person should stop troubling us. Not surprisingly, older people with significant visual losses perceive themselves as a burden to others.

Reactions to failing vision on the part of the affected person can include the following:

○ Disbelief and denial, with a reluctance to take action that might ameliorate or even prevent further losses, like using eye drops in glaucoma or considering cataract extraction.
○ Pining for lost function, with preoccupation with the visual past, anxiety symptoms and emotional lability, irritability and anger.
○ Subsequent depression, as a kind of mourning for the lost self.
○ Resolution and accommodation to the impairment, sometimes related to events like preparing a meal that demonstrate self-sufficiency and increase self-esteem.

Given the potential for grief at loss of visual function, it is hardly surprising that one in three older people identified as visually impaired in one community survey did not take up the specialist assessment offered to them.

The role of general practice

How can the primary care team begin to identify those at risk from such complex impairments? There is no evidence from randomised controlled trials that screening for asymptomatic eye disease in older populations results in improved vision. This may be due to the identification of numbers of people with reduced perceptions of need or concerns about costs of glasses, as well as to long waiting lists for treatments like cataract surgery (Smeeth & Iliffe 1998). A strategy for identifying those individuals with tractable (amenable to treatment) eye disease is needed, and this is likely to depend on opportunistic assessment, as well as targeted attention to 'at risk' groups. The practice nurse who removed Mr. V's sutures is in a good position to ask about changes in his eyesight but will need some reliable way of interpreting the answers, and perhaps a reliable but simple test to get an objective measure of change. Measurement of visual acuity alone is unlikely to be sufficient, since many older people with good acuity are effectively visually impaired in performing everyday tasks involving low and changing light levels, glare and low contrast (Brabyn et al 2001). We will return to the problems of measuring acuity, after recognising that self-reported visual function may be a better way to assess visual impairment.

However, the reliability of simple questions is variable. The screening questions of the kind advocated by the Royal College of General Practitioners are poor at detecting clinically significant reductions in visual acuity, as shown in Table 10.1.

The middle question appears to be more sensitive than the others, but it was asked of people who had already identified themselves as having some kind of visual problem. By combining the questions, the sensitivity of identifying visual acuity of < 6/12 increases to 86%.

Testing distance acuity with a Snellen chart is quick and easy, and 95% of general practitioners have such charts. The test is not reliable if not used at the correct distance and in poor illumination, and will not detect uncorrected presbyopia, for which reading charts are needed. Pin-hole testing with the Snellen chart can help distinguish refractive from non-refractive visual impairment. Looking for a red reflex using an ophthalmoscope is also easy and brief, and can be used to identify individuals with cataracts.

Table 10.1: Screening for visual impairment

Question	Visual acuity comparison	Sensitivity	Specificity
Do you have difficulty seeing distant objects? (with spectacles if you have them)	<6/18	28%	93%
Are you able to recognise a friend across the road?	<6/18	64%	48%
Two questions: • Have you ever worn glasses or contact lenses? • Do you have trouble with your vision even when wearing glasses or contact lenses?	Between 6/12 and 6/18	34%	84%

Derived from Smeeth 1998.

So who should have their vision assessed in primary care, and by whom? The lack of evidence of benefit from screening asymptomatic older people means that a whole-population approach cannot be recommended. Those who present with symptoms should be assessed, using a combination of questions, a check for a red reflex, and acuity measurement with use of a pin-hole. Mr. V did present with a symptom ('I did not see it coming') and so should be counted as symptomatic and assessed. Three-quarters of older people who fall and are admitted to hospital are likely to have remediable visual defects, and so this group (in fact, any recurrent fallers) should be assessed. Although it is not clear what level of visual acuity should act as a threshold for referral for specialist review, any symptoms apparently impairing daily life, or putting the individual at risk, should be investigated further.

KEY LEARNING POINTS— VISUAL IMPAIRMENT

○ Practitioners should focus assessment of vision on older patients with symptomatic eye disease and on those who fall repeatedly.

○ Assessments should include a combination of questions, visual acuity measurement, pin-hole testing and red reflex testing.

○ Assessment should be done before referring for specialist review.

○ Follow up with support for those found to be profoundly visually impaired.

Mrs. H took great care to wear her hearing aid every day, even when she had no visitors, but rarely fitted the battery. The district nurse who was visiting her to dress her leg ulcer found this out, and asked her why she did this. Her reply was: 'If I wear the aid people stop going on at me about using it, and if I leave the batteries out I don't hear the horrible hissing' (Iliffe 2000).

Tutorial — hearing impairment

Mrs. H is not alone in any aspect of her problem. Deafness is a common problem of later life, but seemingly not as damaging to the individual as visual loss, so that remedial action is not taken as frequently and as effectively as it might be. The stigma associated with deafness, that prompts people to want to avoid using an aid and manufacturers to concentrate on making aids discrete, seems disproportional to the impairment, perhaps because the invisibility of deafness makes others attribute the unresponsiveness of the deaf person to disinterest, rudeness or stupidity. Although patients may ask their general practitioner for advice about what to do about their hearing problems, deafness can be a difficult problem to correct. Nevertheless, there is a case for early detection and intervention in primary care, which we will now explore.

About a quarter of individuals aged 65 and over report a problem with their hearing, and one-third have measurable hearing loss (Mulrow & Lichtenstein 1991). It is estimated that 8.7 million adults in Britain have some degree of deafness, of whom 75% are aged 65 or over (Roper & Setchfield 1998). Unlike visual loss, a single pathological process accounts for this common impairment, for the great majority have presbycusis, a gradual and progressive bilateral high frequency sensorineural loss that impairs understanding of speech. Presbycusis is related to the physiological ageing process, but may be worsened by other medical conditions, including:

○ diabetes

○ hypothyroidism

○ hyperlipidaemia

○ hypertension

- ischaemic heart disease
- stroke
- arthritis
- chronic lung disease
- renal disease
- viral and bacterial infections.

Behavioural and environmental factors, like alcohol consumption or noise exposure, also seem to exacerbate presbycusis, and some drugs (aspirin, diuretics like frusemide and bumetanide, and antibiotics) are implicated as causes of hearing loss. The mechanisms behind these associations are unclear, and it is not known whether optimising the management of diabetes or COPD, for example, makes any difference to hearing function or the progress of presbycusis.

These associations have two consequences for the deaf person and the doctor. The first is that the major and serious pathologies will get all the attention, and that hearing loss will fall off the agenda of consultations about diabetes management, control of COPD or cholesterol reduction, for example. The second is that the new focus on these clinical problems will allow us to add a question about hearing to the end of the routine reviews of long-term conditions, perhaps using the kind of self-completed questionnaire that we discuss below.

Whilst presbycusis accounts for the great majority of hearing loss in older people, it is not the only cause of hearing problems and symptoms, and needs to be distinguished from:

- conductive hearing loss sometimes due to ear infection, and rarely to tumours of the middle ear
- sensorineural loss, due to Ménière's disease or an acoustic neuroma.

Sudden onset of sensorineural deafness or unilateral symptoms warrant further investigation and referral to an ENT clinic, whilst bilateral sensorineural loss uncomplicated by infection, fluctuation, persistent tinnitus or vertigo may be best investigated in an audiology clinic after an appropriate work-up (see below). The appearance of high street hearing clinics, equivalent to opticians, may make the correction of hearing loss easier and prompt more people to seek advice from their general practitioners.

The standard criteria for screening are met by hearing loss, up to a point. The burden of disease and disability is significant, there are brief screening tests, and interventions can be effective. However, patient concordance with screening and intervention is not great, and the health service is probably unable to cope with the volume of demand for assessment and remedial action. The more we investigate this, the more complex the problems appear and the more we learn about the relationship between impairment and disability.

Clinical burden

Deafness is associated with diminished sense of wellbeing, and has adverse effects on physical, cognitive, emotional, behavioural and social functioning. Deaf older people report greater limitations in their activity compared with their peers with normal hearing, and make more demands on medical services. The reasons for withdrawal from activities (particularly social activities) are obvious, but the reason for increased use of medical care is less so. The risks of deafness are higher in working class populations, probably because of occupational noise exposure or exposure to organotoxic solvents. One lesson that could be learned from these associations is that a GP's threshold for assessment of hearing should be low in general practice, particularly with older people in industrial (or former industrial) areas.

The impact of hearing loss on older people seems sufficient to produce communication difficulties and social and (sometimes) emotional isolation, although this withdrawal may be accepted as the 'least worst' option (as with Mrs. H above) and be accepted by others as a normal adaptation to ageing. Deafness may contribute to the onset of depression if it is experienced as a major loss, and also to the development of cognitive impairment, although these are not consistent findings. Depressed and cognitively impaired individuals are more likely to report hearing impairment that is not detectable on objective examination. However, although the burden of deafness appears to be significant for older people, it lacks the persuasive power of visual loss because it does not impact forcefully on services and produces changes in behaviour that can be attributed very readily to 'old age'.

Screening tests

As with visual loss, no single, brief screening instrument is sensitive or specific enough to be used routinely in population screening. We advocate a step-wise approach, asking simple questions first as part of a brief check-list for identifying unmet need in older people (Iliffe et al 2004). The initial question is: 'Do you have any difficulty with your hearing?', and this can be supplemented by questions about hearing in noisy environments, turning radios or televisions up loud enough to provoke criticism or complaint. Whisper tests, the finger rub test and use of a tuning fork have some value in the first stage of an assessment in alerting the clinician to potential deafness in the patient, although they are not reliable enough when used alone. An audiometry examination, or use of a portable audioscope, is appropriate given that the latter's sensitivity in detecting failure to hear a 40 db tone range from 87–96%, with specificities of 70–90%, and good repeatability. A self-assessment questionnaire is a useful adjunct to audiometry, the most extensively tested and widely used being the Hearing Handicap Inventory for the Elderly (Screening version) (Lichtenstein et al 1988) (HHIE-S; see Box 10.1). This is what we would recommend for use as part of chronic disease management. A 'no' response scores zero, 'sometimes' scores 2 and 'yes' scores 4. A score of less than 10 indicates no handicap, and greater than 24 indicates moderate to severe handicap. Although religious belief and church attendance are still important in older cohorts in the UK, the question on attendance at religious services (derived from American social habits) may need modification for British populations.

BOX 10.1: Hearing Handicap Inventory for the Elderly (Screening version)[†]

- Does a hearing problem cause you to feel embarrassed when you meet new people?
- Does a hearing problem cause you to feel frustrated when talking to members of your family?
- Do you have difficulties hearing when someone talks in a whisper?
- Do you feel handicapped by a hearing problem?
- Does a hearing problem cause you difficulty when visiting friends, relatives or neighbours?
- Does a hearing problem cause you to attend religious services less often than you would like?
- Does a hearing problem cause you to have arguments with family members?
- Does a hearing problem cause you to have difficulty when listening to television or radio?

BOX 10.1: Hearing Handicap Inventory for the Elderly
(Screening version)[†]—continued

- Do you feel that any difficulty with your hearing limits/hampers your personal or social life?
- Does a hearing problem cause you difficulty when in a restaurant with family or friends?

[†]From Ventry I, Weinstein B. Identification of elderly with hearing problems. ASHA 1983; 25:37–42. Reproduced by permission of the American Speech and Hearing Association © 1983.

Does treatment work?

There are no randomised controlled trials of interventions in the community to guide practitioners about the effectiveness of treatments, but before-and-after and case-control community studies and RCTs in selected populations have demonstrated improved psychological and social functioning, better communication and fewer depression symptoms after hearing aid fitting.

Uptake of hearing aids depends on their cost to the patient, and their capacity to induce embarrassment by drawing attention to the handicap. Actual use may be determined by adverse effects like significant amplification of background noise. According to one American community study, about one in five of those who might benefit from sound amplification use or have tried hearing aids, with greatest use among those with greatest disability and the most educated. However, it does not seem possible as yet to identify those who are most likely to take up and use remediable services. Adapting to hearing aid use does not appear easy for many older people, so correct fitting of aids, training in listening strategies and communication techniques, and continuing support and counselling for the deaf patient are essential, even if new digital and programmable technologies make aids easier to use.

KEY LEARNING POINTS— HEARING IMPAIRMENT

○ Use simple tests to identify conductive disorders, supplementing a history that includes noise exposure and drug use.

○ Respond to clinical suspicion of deafness in older patients with a self-completion questionnaire, like the HHIE-S, followed by audiometry/audioscope assessment.

○ Include the HHIE-S in the routine review of older people who fall into chronic disease management programmes.

○ Refer to audiology or ENT according to findings.

○ Arrange follow-up and support of hearing aid users.

References

Brabyn J, Schneck M, Haegerstrom-Portnoy G, Lott L. The Smith-Kettlewell Institute longitudinal study of vision function and its impact on the elderly: an overview. Optom Vis Sci 2001; 78(5); 264–269.

Brown MM, Brown CG, Sharma S, Busbee B. Quality of life associated with visual loss: a time trade-off utility analysis comparison with medical health states. Ophthalmol 2003; 110(6):1076–1081.

Frost A, Eachus J, Sparrow J, Peters TJ, Hopper C, Davey-Smith G, Frankel S. Vision-related quality of life impairment in an elderly UK population: associations with age, sex, social class and material deprivation. Eye 2001; 15(Pt6):739–744.

Iliffe S, Drennan V. Primary care for older people. Oxford: Oxford University Press; 2000; 129.

Iliffe S, Lenihan P, Orrell M, Walters K,Drennan V, SeeTai S, SPICE Research Team. The development of a short instrument to identify common unmet needs in older people in general practice Br J Gen Pract 2004; 54(509):914–918.

Lichtenstein MJ, Bess FH, Logan SA. Diagnostic performance of the Hearing Handicap Inventory for the elderly (screening version) against different definitions of hearing loss. Ear Hear 1988; 9(4):208–211.

Mulrow CD, Lichtenstein MJ. Screening for hearing impairment in the elderly: rationale and strategy. J Gen Intern Med 1991; 6:249–258.

Roper TA, Setchfield N. Diagnosis and management of impaired hearing. Geriatric Medicine November 1998: 49–52.

Smeeth L. Assessing the likely effectiveness of screening older people for impaired vision in primary care. Fam Pract 1998; 15 Suppl 1:S24–29.

Smeeth L, Iliffe S. Effectiveness of screening older people for impaired vision in community settings: systematic review of evidence from randomised controlled trials. BMJ 1998; 316:660–663.

van der Pols JC, Bates CJ, McGraw PV, Thompson JR, Reacher M, Prentice A, Finch S. Visual acuity measurements in a national sample of British elderly people. Br J Ophthalmol 2000; 84(2):165–170.

Waller JA. Health status and motor vehicle crashes. New Eng J Med 1991; 324:54–55.

Wormald RP, Wright LA, Courtney P, Beaumont B, Haines AP. Visual problems in the elderly population and implications for services. BMJ 1992; 304: 1226–1229.

CHAPTER 11

The older patient with stroke

CASE HISTORY

Mrs. ST calls the GP surgery at 10 o'clock in the morning sounding very worried and upset. She says she thinks her husband has had a stroke. The receptionist puts the call through to the GP on duty straight away. Mrs. ST explains to the GP that her husband, who is 79, had been well when he got up that morning but after breakfast he had fallen on his way from the kitchen to the living room and now is really not himself. While speaking to her on the phone the GP checks the patient's records and sees that he is an ex-smoker with long-standing hypertension. He has had one transient ischaemic attack a year ago and is on bendroflumethiazide, atenolol and aspirin.

The doctor ascertains over the phone that Mr. ST is conscious but drowsy and a little confused. He is not in pain but has weakness in his right arm and leg, and difficulty in speaking. He has not been inconti-nent. The GP tries to calm Mrs. ST down by explaining that while this could be a stroke it could also possibly be a passing event like he had last year. He says that if she can bring him to the practice he will see him straight away, otherwise he will visit him at home as soon as morning surgery finishes. Mrs. ST doesn't feel he could come in so the GP agrees to visit as soon as he can get there.

When the GP arrives he finds Mr. ST sitting in an armchair with obvious droop on the right side of his face. He clearly recognises the doctor but when he tries to speak his words are garbled. The doctor asks him some closed questions requiring only nods or shakes of the head in response. He is able to understand and answer these. He has an irregular pulse at 90 beats per minute, his blood pressure is 160/100. There is no evidence of head injury and his pupils react nor-mally and equally. There is obvious weakness in the right upper and lower limbs with decreased tone, increased reflexes and reduced sen-sation compared to the left side. No carotid bruits can be heard.

The GP thinks a stroke is the most likely diagnosis. The irregular pulse is a new sign and is probably atrial fibrillation. He tells Mr. and Mrs. ST his concerns. Mrs. ST doesn't want her husband to go to hospital unless he really has to. She can look after him with the GP's help. The doctor decides to discuss the situation with the geriatric registrar on call at the hospital. The registrar agrees that this sounds like a cerebral hemisphere stroke but she explains that he should be seen for basic investigation if not CT scan to confirm the diagnosis. Also if he is in AF this should be treated as soon as possible. She agrees to see him that day in casualty. The GP explains to Mr. and Mrs. ST that it is important for him to go to hospital for at least a few days. Aware that many patients get depressed after a stroke he tells Mr. ST he must think positively and that there is every hope that his problems will improve at least to some extent. He arranges transport to take Mr. and Mrs. ST to the hospital and writes a letter for them to take providing Mr. ST's medical and social history and details of his current medication.

At the hospital Mr. ST is seen by the specialist registrar in elderly medicine who records:

'Pulse rate of 86 per minute, irregular, with apex rate of 112 beats per minute. Blood pressure 165/100 mmHg. Normal first and second heart sounds plus a very short mid-systolic murmur at the apex. Right facial weakness, reduced tone with reduced power (3/5) in the right arm and right leg, associated with exaggerated reflexes and extensor plantar response, reduced sensation to touch and pinprick but with evidence of sensory neglect or inattention. Swallows normally.'

Based on these clinical findings the specialist registrar makes a diagnosis of cerebral infarction presumed secondary to atrial fibrillation and outlines the following plan for the next 48 hours:

Investigations

Full blood count, urea and electrolytes, blood glucose, cardiac enzymes, liver function tests, TSH, cholesterol, electrocardiograph, chest X-ray, CT scan of brain and an echocardiograph.

Management

Start digoxin according to usual dosage regimen. Aim to slow down the ventricular rate below 90 beats per minute. Start aspirin 300 mg a day. Provide graduated compression stockings to prevent venous thrombosis, and refer to physiotherapist, OT and speech and language therapist for assessment. Nursing team to continue four-hourly stroke observations.

Progress over the next 48 hours

All haematological and biochemical investigations including random glucose and TSH come back normal. ECG reveals voltage changes suggestive of mild left ventricular hypertrophy, atrial fibrillation with a rate of 116 per minute with t wave changes in leads 1, AvL, V4 to V6. CT scan reveals a middle cerebral artery infarct with no surrounding oedema.

Assessment by speech and language therapist (SALT) reveals mild delay in swallow with little risk of aspiration. The physiotherapist assesses motor and sensory function and advises the nurses on positioning and handling, while the occupational therapist assesses Mr. ST's ability to carry out activities of daily living and cognition. Assessments by all the therapists suggest that Mr. ST has good potential for recovery but that his frustration, his low mood and his desire to improve quickly are likely to hamper his rehabilitation.

Following these assessments, the multidisciplinary team agrees on short-term goals, however at the team meeting two days later it is decided that it would be in the best interests of Mr. ST if ongoing rehabilitation was to take place in his own home. Referral to the community rehabilitation team is made while the social worker arranges to meet Mr. and Mrs. ST to discuss the support and services they would like to have during the next few weeks. In the meantime the specialist registrar telephones Mr. ST's GP to inform him of the plan for rehabilitation at home. They agree that the GP will visit him at home in relation to his BP, atrial fibrillation and low mood and frustration, while the specialist registrar arranges a follow-up in the day hospital after an echocardiograph has been performed.

Mr. ST makes steady progress at home and by the time of his day hospital assessment 10 days after discharge he is able to walk independently with the aid of one stick. The echocardiograph has revealed a dilated left atrium, mild-to-moderate mitral regurgitation with fairly good ventricular function. The specialist registrar discusses all results with Mr. and Mrs. ST and considers with them the benefits and risks of warfarin and aspirin for his atrial fibrillation. Mr. ST decides not to take warfarin but to continue with aspirin. The specialist registrar writes to the GP outlining the decision made by Mr. ST and recommends regular BP assessment while a further assessment of his functional status is arranged for six months' time in the day hospital.

LEARNING POINTS FROM CASE HISTORY

- Patients with stroke should be referred to hospital for assessment and basic investigations, including CT scan.
- Although stroke is a clinical syndrome, confirmation of diagnosis requires CT scan.
- Involvement of MDT is essential for assessment and management of rehabilitation in hospital and in the community.
- Following discharge, the patient should be seen by GP to ensure that risk factors for stroke are being managed/controlled appropriately.

Tutorial — stroke

Definition

The World Health Organisation has defined stroke as a syndrome of rapidly developing clinical signs of focal (or global) disturbance of cerebral function, with symptoms lasting for 24 hours or longer or leading to death, with no apparent cause other than vascular origin. This includes subarachnoid haemorrhage but excludes TIA, subdural haemorrhage and/or infarction caused by infection or tumour.

Incidence/prevalence

Stroke is a common illness of older people, with a prevalence rate of 5 per 1000. One in four men and one in five women will have stroke if they live to 85 years. As a pathology, it is the third most common cause of death, with a 28-day fatality of 20–28% and a one-year fatality of between 34–41%. At any one time, about 20% of hospital beds are occupied by patients with stroke, and 4–6% of the health service budget is spent on managing stroke.

In recent years, three important publications have appeared outlining the standards of care required for stroke patients in the UK. These are:

National Clinical Guidelines prepared by the Intercollegiate Working Party for stroke organised by the Royal College of Physicians of London (2004).

The Consensus statement by the Royal College of Physicians of Edinburgh (2000).

The National Service Framework for Older People (DoH 2001).

Stroke syndromes

Cerebral infarction can be divided into four syndromes, according to the circulation pathway involved. The first three involve the anterior (carotid) circulation, whilst the fourth involves the posterior (vertebrobasilar) circulation. These are characterised as follows:

TACS (total anterior circulation syndrome): higher cortical dysfunction (dysphasia or visuospatial neglect), homonymous hemianopia and hemiplegia and/or sensory deficit involving at least two of face, arm and leg.

PACS (partial anterior circulation syndrome): two of the three components of TACS, higher dysfunction alone or motor/sensory deficit more restricted than those classified as lacunar events.

LACS (lacunar syndromes)—pure motor, pure sensory, sensorimotor or ataxic hemiplegia.

POCS (posterior circulation syndrome): homonymous hemianopia alone, crossed cranial nerve palsies (e.g. Weber's syndrome), cerebellar syndrome without long tract signs, bilateral motor/sensory deficit.

The prognosis for these stroke subtypes is very different. More than 50% of patients with TACS are dead one year after their stroke, and the majority of those who survive a TACS will remain dependent on care to a greater or lesser degree. In contrast, death following a lacunar event is uncommon (less than 10% at one year), and the majority of these patients will regain full independence.

Treatment of acute stroke

There is now good evidence that thrombolytic treatment with tissue plasminogen activator (tPA) given within three to six hours improves outcome, but this is associated with substantial increase in cerebral haemorrhage within the first two weeks. The updated National Stroke Guidelines recommend that thrombolytic treatment with alteplase should be given provided that:

○ it is administered within three hours of onset of symptoms unless as part of clinical trial

○ haemorrhage has been definitely excluded

○ the NINDS criteria has been met

○ the patient is in a centre registered with Safe Implementation of Thrombolysis in Stroke Monitoring Study (SITS–MOST).

The International Stroke Trial and the Chinese Acute Stroke Trial which included nearly 40 000 patients noted that aspirin produced 6% reduction in odds of death or dependency. National guidelines now recommend that aspirin should be given in a dosage of 300 mg as soon as possible after the onset of stroke if a diagnosis of haemorrhage is considered unlikely. Thereafter, aspirin (50–30 mg) should be continued indefinitely until an alternative antiplatelet therapy is started. In those receiving thrombolysis, aspirin should be delayed for 24 hours.

The European Stroke Study has also shown that a combination of aspirin and modified-release dipyridamole may be slightly more effective than aspirin. NICE recommends this combination for a period of 2 years from the most recent event (ischaemic stroke or TIA). In those with intolerance (including hypersensitivity) to aspirin, it is recommended that clopidogrel 75 mg per day can be substituted.

Other components of immediate management include:

○ maintenance of hydration

○ treatment of hyperglycaemia, if present

○ treatment of pyrexia

○ oxygen if saturation is low.

Early complications of stroke

○ Abnormal tone, contractures, pressure sores and pneumonia—the risk of these early complications associated with stroke can all be minimised by use of patient positioning and pressure-relieving cushions and mattresses.

○ Venous thromboembolism—best prevented by use of compression stockings.

○ Urinary and faecal incontinence—both are common in the early stages and it is essential that these are managed as part of rehabilitation. If incontinence cannot be cured, adequate continence aids and services should be organised prior to discharge.

○ Depression is common after stroke, with symptoms of crying, hopelessness, lack of motivation, poor appetite, etc. It often responds well to antidepressant therapy.

○ Speech problems—dysphasia, dysarthria, and articulatory dyspraxia—all require accurate assessment and management by a speech and language therapist.

Late complications of stroke

○ Spasticity—managed by physical treatment and/or antispasticity drugs.

○ Pain—this may arise from pre-existing conditions, such as osteoarthritis or due to brain damage resulting from stroke (central pain), which may require tricyclic antidepressant therapy or carbamazepine.

Secondary prevention

1. ANTICOAGULATION IN PATIENTS WITH ATRIAL FIBRILLATION

National Stroke Guidelines in the UK recommend anticoagulation (warfarin with suggested INR of 2-3) in cases of AF (persistent or paroxysmal, valvular or non-valvular), prosthetic heart valves or within three months of MI, but the optimal timing for initiating treatment after the acute stroke is unresolved. A suggested waiting period of two weeks covered by aspirin is included in the guidelines.

While warfarin has been shown to reduce the risk of stroke by 62% compared to placebo, aspirin has been shown to reduce the risk by 22%.

2. BLOOD PRESSURE MANAGEMENT FOLLOWING STROKE

There is currently no randomised data available on the management of blood pressure during the acute phase of stroke, when BP is often raised. Lowering BP acutely is associated with poor prognosis unless there are signs of malignant hypertension, or aortic dissection with renal impairment. Over the medium term it is recommended that BP is treated if at four weeks post-CVA the value exceeds 140/85 mmHg in non-diabetics and >130/80 in diabetics.

Two recent studies (HOPE and PROGRESS) have shown that use of ACE inhibitors, ramipril (HOPE 2000) and perindopril (PROGRESS 2001), can significantly reduce the recurrence of vascular events, including myocardial infarction and death. The reduction is seen not only in known hypertensive patients but also in normotensive patients. See Table 11.1 for a list of hypotensive drugs used in stroke prevention.

3. LOWERING CHOLESTEROL AFTER STROKE

Although there are currently no randomised control trials on the effect of lowering cholesterol following stroke, it is recommended that those with total cholesterol of >3.5 mmol/l and particularly those who have clinical history or signs of ischaemic heart disease, peripheral vascular disease or diabetes should be treated with these agents. See Table 11.2 for a list of lipid-lowering drugs used in stroke prevention.

4. THE ROLE OF CAROTID ENDARTERECTOMY

Carotid endarterectomy has a role in preventing stroke in patients who have severe stenosis (i.e. >70 %) as soon as they are fit for surgery, and also those with less severe stenosis who are considered to be at high risk of further stroke, i.e. those with frequent TIAs, cerebral rather than ocular symptoms, ulcerated rather than smooth stenosis. Success of this operation is dependent upon the experience of the surgeon, and therefore it is important that surgery is carried out in a specialised centre. Data suggests that the benefit of endarterectomy persists for three years after operation.

Prognosis following stroke

It is reasonably accurate to think in terms of a rule of thirds. Around one-third of patients with stroke die in the first month after the event. Approximately, two-thirds of those who survive a year are able to live independently, while a third of these survivors are disabled requiring help with basic activities of daily living.

Table 11.1: Hypotensive drugs used in stroke prevention

Group of drug	Action	Main side effects
Diuretics, e.g. bendroflumethiazide, indapamide	Unknown, although main long-term effect is via reduction in PVR	Serious: rare Mild: hypokalaemia, hyponatraemia, hypercholesterolaemia, skin rashes, pancreatitis, blood dyscrasias
Beta-blockers, e.g. bisoprolol, carvedilol, metoprolol	Antagonism to peripheral beta-receptors	Bradycardia, heart failure, general weakness, depression Raise triglycerides and lower HDL cholesterol
ACE inhibitors, e.g. enalapril, ramipril, perindopril	Reduce the conversion of angiotensin I to angiotensin II by ACE inhibition	Cough (10–15%), renal impairment (particularly in those with renal artery stenosis), first-dose hypotension (rare)
Calcium-channel blockers, e.g. amlodipine, diltiazem, isradipine	Reduce PVR through blocking calcium channels	Headache, flushing, palpitations, fluid retention, heart block
Alpha-blockers, e.g. doxazosin	Selectively block the alpha-1-adrenoreceptors	Hypotension, palpitations
Angiotensin II inhibitors, e.g. losartan, valsartan irbesartan	Block angiotensin II receptors	Cough but less than ACE inhibitors Renal impairment as for ACE-I

Table 11.2: Lipid-lowering drugs used in stroke prevention

Drug	Dose	Side-effects
Simvastatin	10 mg at night adjusted at 4-week intervals	Headache, diarrhoea flatulence, abdominal pain, nausea, vomiting, myalgia/myositis (stop therapy if creatinine kinase is elevated [>5×])
Atorvastatin	10 mg at night adjusted at 4-week intervals	As above
Pravastatin	10 mg at night adjusted at 4-week intervals to maximum dose of 40 mg/day	As above

Although it is difficult to make an accurate assessment of prognosis, there are several well known markers of poorer prognosis and these include:

○ area involved by stroke (survival in TACS is 60% whereas it is nearly 85% in PACS and 90% in LACS)
○ pre-stroke dependency
○ presence of visuospatial dysfunction
○ initially reduced conscious level
○ impaired mobility/severe hemiplegia
○ presence of urinary incontinence.

Advice for patients following stroke

It is important not only to provide accurate information on stroke, including the risk of further stroke, but to ensure that the patient and his or her carers understand the common aspects of the impact of stroke, e.g. effects on mobility and communication, tiredness, loss of confidence and depression. All areas of prevention should be explained in positive terms. This discussion should include advice on diet, smoking, alcohol, exercise and reasons for any medication prescribed. Elderly patients and partners may be shy to ask so it is worth remembering to reassure that sexual activity can be resumed after stroke without any known risk.

Driving following stroke

Patients who were driving before their stroke should be advised that this is not allowed for one month after any stroke or TIA, and that their ability to drive will be dependent upon their own level of recovery. There is no need to notify DVLA **unless** there is residual neurological deficit one month after the episode, in particular visual field defects, cognitive defects and impaired limb function. Minor limb weakness alone will not require notification unless restriction to certain types of vehicle or vehicles with adapted controls is needed. Epileptic attacks occurring at the time of a stroke/TIA or in the ensuing 24 hours may be treated as 'provoked' for licensing purposes in the absence of any previous seizure history or previous cerebral pathology.

Tutorial — transient ischaemic attacks (TIAs)

Definition of TIA

Transient ischaemic attack is a syndrome of sudden onset with focal neurological loss (cerebral or monocular) of presumed vascular origin, lasting less than 24 hours.

Typical features of TIA include:

○ acute onset
○ focal symptoms and signs, e.g. hemiparesis, sensory changes, amaurosis, dysphasia.
○ recovery within 24 hours.

Symptoms that are **rarely** part of TIA include:

○ general light-headedness
○ vertigo
○ dizziness
○ 'funny turn'
○ drowsiness
○ confusion
○ unexplained collapse
○ syncope
○ incontinence
○ general weakness
○ headaches
○ tingling.

Guidelines on management of TIA (Fig. 11.1)

National Stroke Guidelines recommend that patients first seen in the community with TIA should be assessed and investigated in a specialist neurovascular clinic within seven days of onset. They do not need admission unless:

○ the patient cannot be seen in a specialised neurovascular clinic within one week

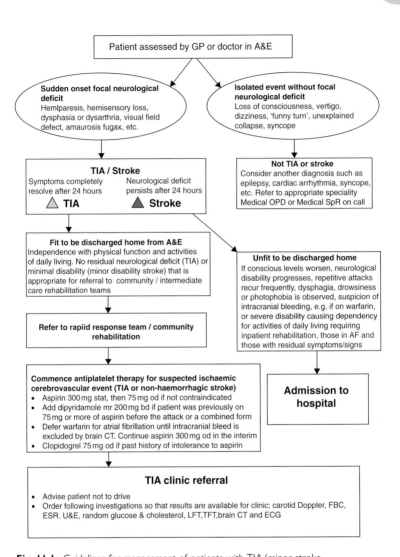

Fig. 11.1: Guidelines for management of patients with TIA/minor stroke.

○ an underlying cause requiring urgent treatment is suspected

○ patient has more than one TIA within a short period (crescendo TIA).

Management in the community

Although national guidance on referral to hospital is clear, general practitioners can appropriately:

○ Offer lifestyle advice on low salt, weight reduction (if indicated), alcohol limits, exercise and smoking.

○ Start aspirin 50–300 mg a day. If already on aspirin prior to TIA, then add dipyridamole SR 200 mg Bd. Those who have intolerance to aspirin should be prescribed clopidogrel 75 mg daily.

○ Order the following investigations: full blood count, ESR, urea and electrolytes, random glucose, cholesterol, liver function tests and thyroid function tests.

○ Check BP and start treatment if indicated (see above for stroke).

Management in the hospital

Management in hospital by a specialist in stroke will include full assessment and investigations to confirm the diagnosis, and to treat/correct possible factors contributing to the TIAs. Investigations will include baseline haematological tests, biochemistry (including cholesterol and random glucose), CT brain scan and carotid Doppler.

Management will naturally take into account the actions already taken by the primary care physician and results of investigations. It will include review of:

1. Antiplatelet therapy (see above).

2. Blood pressure management (Table 11.1)—if a patient is not on any treatment and lifestyle has not managed to lower BP then the patient should be started on a thiazide diuretic or an ACE-inhibitor such as ramipril or perindopril, or preferably a combination of both, unless these are contraindicated with a target BP of 140/85 in non-diabetics and 135/80 in diabetics.

3. Cholesterol (Table 11.2)—lower cholesterol with diet and a statin with an aim to lower total cholesterol below 5 mmol/l or LDL-C to below 3 mmol/l.

4. Atrial fibrillation—if present consider anticoagulation with warfarin with target INR of 2.0–3.0 after CT scan has excluded intracerebral bleed.

5. Result of carotid Doppler examination—those with a symptomatic internal carotid artery stenosis of >70% and who are otherwise fit should be referred to a vascular surgeon for consideration of carotid endarterectomy. Carotid artery angiography or MRI angiography is required prior to surgery. The former carries a small but distinct risk of inducing a stroke. Carotid endarterectomy has a 1–2% perioperative stroke risk in the most experienced hands but reduces the incidence of stroke by 75% over the next two to three years.

Updated guidelines from the Royal College of Physicians recommend that carotid endarterectomy should be performed as soon as the patient is fit, preferably within two weeks of TIA, since the greatest benefit of surgery is achieved from early surgery with little or no benefit if surgery is delayed beyond three months of TIA.

It should be noted that asymptomatic carotid stenosis is associated with a lower stroke risk and benefit from surgery is not proven.

Prognosis after TIA over four years

Of all patients suffering definite TIA it can be estimated that by four years:

○ 25% have died

○ 25% have suffered stroke

○ 10% have suffered myocardial infarction.

Advice on driving after TIA

Advice on driving after TIA is basically the same as after a stroke. Patients must not drive for at least one month. They may resume driving after this time if the clinical recovery is satisfactory. There is no need to notify DVLA **unless** there is residual neurological deficit one month after the episode, in particular visual field defects, cognitive defects and impaired limb function. Minor limb weakness alone will not require notification unless restriction to certain types of vehicle or vehicles with adapted controls is needed. A driver experiencing multiple TIAs over a short period of time may require three months freedom of further attacks before resuming driving and should notify DVLA.

Tutorial — other causes of stroke

Cerebral venous thrombosis

Occlusion of cerebral veins or dural vein sinuses may present as a stroke syndrome, subarachnoid haemorrhage or as an isolated raised intracranial pressure. Patients at risk of developing this condition are those with prothrombotic tendency, those with ear or nasal sinus infections, those with disseminated malignancy and patients with dehydration. In addition to stroke syndrome, headache is a prominent symptom and may occur several weeks before the stroke. National Stroke Guidelines recommend MRI with MRV as investigations and treatment with heparin.

Cervical arterial dissection

A tear in the intima of carotid or vertebral artery results in thrombus, from which an embolus can lead to TIA or ischaemic stroke. Although it is associated with trauma or abnormal movement of neck (particularly rotation), it can occur spontaneously. It is common in children or younger adults below 50 years of age and should also be considered in patients with Horner's syndrome or evidence of collagen disease. Treatment with anticoagulants is recommended for six months.

Subarachnoid haemorrhage

National Stroke Guidelines recommend:

1. Immediate CT scan if patient has impaired level of consciousness and within 12 hours in all patients.
2. If CT negative, lumbar puncture performed.
3. Once diagnosis is confirmed, give nimodipine 60 mg four-hourly, unless contraindicated.
4. Refer to neurosurgeon immediately.
5. Patients with a strong family history (i.e. one other first-degree relative affected and/or with history of polycystic kidneys) should be advised to ask for a referral for the family to attend a neurovascular specialist for advice.

KEY LEARNING POINTS—STROKE

○ Stroke is defined as a focal neurological deficit of vascular origin, which lasts more than 24 hours. It may be due to cerebral infarction (80%) or haemorrhage (20%).

○ Differential diagnosis should include intercurrent illness with previous stroke, hypoglycaemia and hyperglycaemia, head injury, infection, tumours, migraine, epilepsy, SBE, musculoskeletal injury, e.g. fractured hip or humerus.

○ Aspirin is an important part of initial treatment if haemorrhage is considered unlikely or has been excluded on CT scan.

○ It is a fundamental step in the management of stroke to distinguish between cerebral infarction and haemorrhage, and therefore CT scanning is essential. It also helps to exclude other non-vascular causes of stroke.

○ There is strong evidence that people with stroke are more likely to survive and recover function if admitted promptly and managed by a specialist coordinated stroke team

○ Management, following initial assessment and support, consists of identification and modification of risk factors and intensive rehabilitation using a multidisciplinary approach. This may start in hospital but must be continued in the community.

○ Depression (in patients and carers) is a common consequence of stroke and all health professionals should be aware of this possibility.

○ Patients first seen in the community with TIA should be assessed and investigated in a specialist neurovascular clinic within 7 days of onset. They do not need admission unless:

   i   the patient cannot be seen in a specialised neurovascular clinic within two week

   ii an underlying cause requiring urgent treatment is suspected

   iii patient has more than one TIA within a short period (crescendo TIA).

References

Department of Health. National Service Framework for Older People, 2001.

Heart Outcomes Prevention Evaluation (HOPE) Study Investigators. Effects of ramipril on cardiovascular and microvascular outcomes in people with diabetes mellitus. Lancet 2000; 355(9200):253–259.

PROGRESS Collaborative Group. Randomised trial of a perindopril-based blood-pressure-lowering regimen among 6105 individuals with previous stroke or transient ischaemic attack. Lancet 2001; 358(9287):1033–1041.

Royal College of Physicians of Edinburgh. Consensus Statement (updated November 2000).

Royal College of Physicians. National Clinical Guidelines for Stroke. 2nd edn. London: Clinical Effectiveness and Evaluation Unit, 2004.

Further reading

Benavente O, Hart RG. Stroke: Part II. Management of acute ischaemic stroke. Am Fam Physician. 1999; 59(10): 2828–2834.

Further information

Safe Implementation of Thrombolysis in Stroke. International Stroke Thrombolysis Register (SITS–ISTR). **www.acutestroke.com.**

CHAPTER 12

The older patient
with depression

Mr. DA, aged 76, rarely visits his GP but goes to the surgery one day complaining that he has no energy and is sleeping badly. He wakes frequently at night and feels weary when he gets up in the morning. He has lost his appetite. His wife died three years ago following a stroke. Whilst he volunteers that he does not get out and enjoy himself these days, he is adamant that he is not depressed.

Tutorial — depression

Depression is the commonest psychiatric disorder in later life, with population studies showing that 10–15% of the population aged 65 or more suffer with significant depressive symptoms. Older patients in general practice have higher levels of psychological morbidity than do population samples, and this morbidity is often not recognised. The housebound are twice as likely to experience depression than more mobile older people. Populations living in sheltered accommodation may have an even higher prevalence of depression, closer to one in four individuals. Mental ill-health caries a stigma of weakness or madness that makes many reluctant to accept depression as a diagnosis.

Mr. DA's general practitioner will check that he has not got diabetes, hypothyroidism, anaemia or other cause for his symptoms, whilst noting that he does have some of the typical symptoms of a depressive disorder (Box 12.1).

BOX 12.1: Core symptoms of depressive episode[1]

- Depressed mood sustained for at least two weeks (on most days, much of the time) and/or
- Loss of interest or pleasure in usual activities

And/or
- Decreased energy, increased fatigue (in patients who are physically ill this may mean feelings of fatigue even when not attempting exertion); diminished activity

---

BOX 12.1: continued

Other symptoms:
- Suicidal thoughts or behaviour
- Loss of confidence or self-esteem
- Feeling of helplessness
- Inappropriate or excessive guilt
- Feelings of hopelessness or worthlessness
- Avoiding social interactions or going out
- Poor concentration and/or difficulty with memory
- Psychomotor retardation or agitation (restlessness or fidgeting)
- Sleep disturbance
- Reduced appetite with corresponding weight loss.

Mr. DA may feel that his situation is understandable, perhaps even inevitable, because we all loose our family and friends and are own abilities as we age. Mr. DA's GP may agree with this and not want to medicalise everyday sorrows. Where is the boundary between depressive disorders and understandable sadness? We suggest that the following distinguish normal grief, sorrow and unhappiness from depression:

- **Duration:** symptoms are present for at least two weeks.
- **Lack of fluctuation:** occur most days, most of the time.
- **Intensity:** must be of a degree that is definitely not normal for that individual.

Depression, then, is profound, persistent and pervasive which is why Mr. DA has come to see his family doctor.

Under-recognition

Only a small minority of depressed older individuals with significant symptoms receive treatment or referral, even though their general practitioners frequently recognise their depressed state (MacDonald 1986). The severity of the depression and high levels of anxiety seem to be triggers for referral (Eustace et al 2001), but as a whole it seems true to say that depression in later life is underestimated, under-diagnosed and under-treated. Its significance is underestimated despite evidence that:

○ late life depression is associated with disproportionately high rates of suicide and high mortality from all causes

○ depression in later life is associated with high use of both medical and social services

○ depressed older people are more likely to be treated for anxiety (or physical symptoms like pain) than with antidepressants or psychological therapies

○ depression particularly affects those older people caring for others.

There are many reasons for this under-recognition problem, one of them being the complexity of depressive disorders in later life and the difficulty general practitioners face in treating them. Therapeutic interventions depend on a common understanding between general practitioners and specialists of which treatments work for which types of depression, and so an awareness of the taxonomy of depression is the basis for any approach to shared care.

Types of depression

There are three clusters of depressive disorder, different in their severity (essentially, the number of symptoms and their

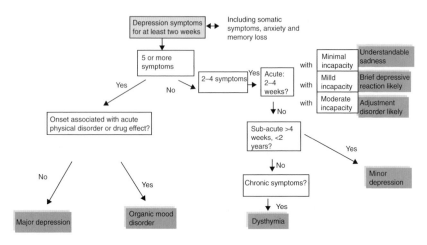

Fig. 12.1 Decision tree for the differential diagnosis of late life depression.

impact) and their duration. Figure 12.1 shows a decision tree to guide practitioners in assessment of depression. This is not an academic exercise, because it guides therapeutic interventions and determines when specialist help should be sought.

Like all taxonomies of disturbances of mental health, this is to some extent arbitrary, and some individuals will not fit the pattern at all. Nevertheless, it works well enough and is memorable. Anyone with five or more depressive symptoms for more than two weeks may have a major depressive disorder, or an organic brain syndrome (from alcohol, drugs or dementia). Those with four or fewer depression symptoms have either dysthymia (symptoms for more than two years), minor depression (symptoms for less than two years) or short-term disturbances in mood and functioning that can be categorised according to their impact on daily life (Fig 12.1).

MAJOR DEPRESSION

Only a minority of those with depressive symptoms have a sufficient number with sufficient severity to warrant the diagnosis of major depression. This type of depression responds better than all others to antidepressant therapy, and timely advice on treatment should be given (see below) along with a recommendation to seek specialist assessment and advice. Organic brain syndromes are likely to have other symptoms alongside features of depression (e.g. memory loss or loss of ability to do everyday tasks) and histories of excess alcohol consumption or long-term medication use (e.g. benzodiazepine dependence). If there are numerous depression symptoms but uncertainties about any possible organic brain disorder, the logical first step is to seek specialist advice and share longer-term management on the basis of a specialist's assessment. Contrast Mr. DA with the following case.

Mr. DB, aged 93, lives alone, supported by home care because of his blindness. He complains that his memory is getting worse, and that he cannot remember people's names or where he has put things. He has become less talkative over the last few weeks, changing from cheerful and interested in his carers' lives and families to being unforthcoming and concerned only with practical things in his everyday life.

Does he have early signs of dementia or is he becoming depressed? Those who complain about memory loss usually do not have dementia, and withdrawal can be a feature of depression. However, 40% of those with early dementia have depression symptoms. Assessment by an old age psychiatrist or geriatrician is needed, ideally before any treatment is initiated.

MINOR DEPRESSION

Most older people have fewer depression symptoms and fall into the category of 'minor depression', in which the appropriateness of the clinical label of depression may be contested by patients and their families and where the effectiveness of treatments is unknown. This form of depression in later life is characterised by variability of symptoms, including prominent features of anxiety, somatisation and an association with disability. It is nebulous enough to have acquired many names — 'demoralisation syndrome', 'dysphoria', 'atypical depression', 'masked depression', 'sub-syndromal depression' amongst others. In epidemiological studies it is about three times more common in older people than major depression and is, therefore, the most common type of depression encountered in primary care. The correlates of minor depression are shown in Box 12.2 and suggest that calling it 'minor' may be a misnomer.

BOX 12.2: 'Minor depression' in the community

- Found among more ill, older people
- Associated with functional impairment, which may wax and wane in synchrony with depressive symptoms
- Associated with cognitive impairment
- Linked to later major depression, as a possible precursor state
- Associated with social and family impairment
- Associated with higher death rates from all causes

Dysthymia

Dysthymia, in the sense of a chronic depressive state, is associated with significant physical impairment. Depression and disability are commonly associated, but the majority of older people with disabilities are not depressed. Nevertheless, disability and depression are risk factors for each other; disabilities can trigger depression, whilst depression can be itself disabling. A study of a large cohort of older people with physical limitations compared depression symptoms and ADL/IADL measures and found a strong contemporaneous effect of changing disability on depressive symptoms, a weaker one-year lagged effect of depression on disability and a weak correlation between the stable components of depression and disability (Ormel et al 2002).

The following case shows how loss of function can promote depression in someone whose coping mechanisms do not allow her to accommodate to her changed ability.

CASE HISTORY 3

Mrs. DC, aged 82, tries to remain physically and mentally active, and likes to garden, although bending and stooping have become increasingly difficult. She gets low back pain which spreads down the front of her thighs, and she cannot walk far because of this but is still driving. To her, the pain is due to arthritis. Her sleep is disturbed by this pain and she asks her GP for sleeping tablets on a regular basis, saying 'it's terrible getting old'. In the past she has had two severe bouts of depression, one in her twenties and another in her mid-fifties; in both cases she was treated in hospital.

The association between poor health and depression appears to be greater for those aged 75 and over and for men, than for 'younger' old people as a whole and for women. Poor health, loss of mobility and depression are linked with loneliness and social isolation. Subjective measures of ill-health like pain or self-rating of health are more strongly related to depression than are more objective measures of illness or disability like the number of chronic diseases or the degree of functional limitation. Nearly a third of older people with four or more medical problems are depressed, compared with one in twenty of those without a significant illness, and the prevalence of depression amongst patients with poor physical health attending their general practitioner is twice that of healthy patients. The difficulty for general practitioners and specialists alike is knowing how best to respond to dysthymia, because as we shall see later the effectiveness of therapies is less certain than with major depression. Consider the next case in the light of this knowledge, and think about the approach you might take to managing the problems it creates; we will return to it.

Mrs. DD, aged 81, has emphysema and type 2 diabetes. Recently she learned that she has a cataract in one eye, after noticing a change in her vision. She gets very short of breath when walking, even on the flat, and stairs are becoming a major problem for her. Her husband died 10 years ago, and her only son died from a brain tumour at the age of 35. She has started cooking classes at the local college, and has one or two friends whom she sees each month. She visits her doctor regularly with lots of vague aches and pains, saying she has 'no get up and go' and that she has 'lived too long'.

There are no right answers, but at the very least Mrs. DD should be offered regular consultations with her GP for supportive and review purposes, and her medical care should be organized carefully to maximize her functional ability. She has a small social network and some outside interests, and she needs to be encouraged to maintain them during her current difficulties. If she experiences her situation in psychological terms, accepting that she is at risk of becoming depressed even if she does not believe she is yet, more formal counselling or CBT should be offered. If her energy loss is impeding daily life or is associated with other biological symptoms (e.g. sleep disturbance, loss of appetite), antidepressant therapy should be offered, using an SSRI. A home visit would provide a lot of information about how she is coping, assuming she would allow it.

Few symptoms and short duration

The short-term depressive disorders (brief depressive reaction, adjustment disorders and 'understandable sadness') are the kind of self-limiting problems that general practitioners deal with all the time. The clinical skill lies in holding the problem and containing the anxiety it generates in the person and those around them until remission begins. The clinical risk lies in not noticing how short-term shades into longer-term, and thinking of a persistent, pervasive grief at the loss of self or others as no more than 'understandable sadness'. Depression can become a semi-permanent state, with waxing and waning of symptoms, making it more of a chronic disease to be managed than an acute illness to be treated.

Prognosis

Depression in later life has a poor prognosis, with a chronic relapsing course (Cole et al 1999). A study from the Netherlands showed that amongst depressed older people attending general practice, a third remitted without relapse after one year, a quarter remitted but relapsed and 40% remained chronically depressed (Beekman et al 1995).

Late-life depression is also associated with higher than expected morbidity, disability and mortality from a wide range of natural causes. One large scale community study has shown that the relative risks of both all-cause mortality and cardiovascular mortality are highest in depressed individuals with established heart disease, but are also elevated in those with no evidence of cardiovascular pathology at entry to the study (Aromaa et al 1994). Depression is one of the main risk factors for sudden death up to one year after myocardial infarction, after adjustment for other risk factors, and also predicts a poorer outcome after life-threatening illness like subarachnoid haemorrhage, pulmonary embolism or bleeding peptic ulcer, even allowing for illness severity (Silverstone 1990).

Depression is the psychiatric condition most often linked to suicide among older adults, and suicide is associated with physical illness in older age groups rather than the substance abuse and personality disorders that characterize younger cohorts. High and rising rates of suicide among older adults (particularly men) are a worldwide phenomenon, and the increasing incidence of depression in recent cohorts portends ominously for future generations of older adults. Most elderly patients who commit suicide have had recent contact with their GP (about a third within the preceding week) and most have major depression. The following indicate higher risk:

- **Demography:** older age and gender (especially old men aged over 80) and isolation.
- **History:** a history of previous attempt(s), evidence of planning such as altering wills and a recent bereavement.
- **Physical factors:** chronic and painful medical disorders, alcohol misuse and abuse of sedatives/hypnotics.
- **Mental state:** suicidal thoughts, plans of suicide, marked agitation (patient is objectively restless and feels inward restlessness), profound hopelessness, feelings of worthlessness, guilt or self-reproach, marked insomnia, marked hypochondriasis and psychotic ideation.

Mr. DE, aged 89, is seen at home by his GP. His home care worker reports that he is very anxious and always seeking reassurance. His wife died two years ago, and nine months ago he had a stroke which left him confined to a wheelchair. He denies being depressed but admits to not enjoying anything, saying 'how would you feel in my position?'. He has difficulty sleeping, has lost weight and refuses meals on wheels because 'they taste awful'. One month ago he started to experience urinary incontinence but says it is 'just part of getting old' and that nothing can be done.

The obvious lessons from this story are that anxiety can mask depression, and that his physical changes suggest either a severe depressive illness or new pathology. Anhedonia is more common than guilt as a dominant symptom in late life depression, but the pattern here (an isolated older man with a significant disability and a new, uncomfortable and embarrassing problem) increases the risk of suicide.

The general practitioner's role

Perhaps the most important role of the GP is to be alert to the possibility of depression in older patients and the fact that it may often be masked. The diagnosis of depression is a clinical one, but detection can be aided by use of some simple screening tools. Probably the best known of these for older people is the Geriatric Depression Scale (GDS). The short (i.e. 15 question) version of this is shown in Box 12.3.

BOX 12.3: Geriatric Depression Scale (short version)	
Choose the best answer for how you have felt over the past week	**Score**
1. Are you basically satisfied with your life?	Yes = 1 point
2. Have you dropped many of your activities and interests?	Yes = 1 point
3. Do you feel that your life is empty	Yes = 1 point
4. Do you often get bored?	Yes = 1 point
5. Are you in good spirits most of the time?	No = 1 point
6. Are you afraid that something bad is going to happen to you?	Yes = 1 point
7. Do you feel happy most of the time?	No = 1 point

BOX 12.3: Geriatric Depression Scale (short version)—continued

8. Do you feel helpless?	Yes = 1 point
9. Do you prefer to stay at home, rather than going out and doing new things?	Yes = 1 point
10. Do you feel you have more problems with memory than others?	Yes = 1 point
11. Do you think it is wonderful to be alive?	No = 1 point
12. Do you feel pretty worthless the way you are now?	Yes = 1 point
13. Do you feel full of energy?	No = 1 point
14. Do you feel that your situation is hopeless?	Yes = 1 point
15. Do you think that most people are better off than you are?	Yes = 1 point
Scoring intervals: 0–4 = no depression, 5–10 = mild depression, 11–15 = severe depression	

Depression in later life requires a long-term commitment to treatment and follow-up in which the general practitioner is likely to be the key clinical worker, even when the initial diagnosis and first treatment plan have been developed by an old-age psychiatrist or geriatrician. The general principles of management of late life depression are these (WPA 1999):

1. **Education.** The most important step is the education of the patient (and care givers) about depression and their involvement in treatment decisions. This means exploring the individual's understanding of their depression, including its causes, and working through any perceptions that may impede efforts to restore normal mood and functioning (e.g. depression as just desserts, or as a moral fault). It may also mean that the general

practitioner has to accept the expertise of the individual, without loosing the critical listening faculties that will pick-up worsening hopelessness and self-destructive thinking.

2. **Treat depression symptoms with the aim of achieving complete remission** (as residual symptoms are a risk factor for chronic depression) but not necessarily 'cure'. Expectations need to be realistic, both in terms of the speed of recovery (mostly slow) and also the prospects for complete and irreversible recovery (which may not happen). An individual who may need long-term (even life-long) antidepressant treatment needs to have that perspective, and not be left expecting rapid changes or no return of symptoms. Of course, older people who have experienced episodes of depression earlier in life may be very familiar with the relapsing nature of this disorder and may need little convincing that it cannot be eradicated from their existence completely. What they may need is the sense that they can go 'into remission'. By its nature, depression erodes optimism, and the very history that might make them (and us) realistic could also breed a sense of hopelessness.

3. **Treat the whole person.** Other physical disorders, including poor vision and hearing deficits, can make the depressed individual more isolated and less capable of helping themselves. Always sign-post the patient to appropriate social care agencies, and review their medication with a view to withdrawing those unnecessary drug treatments that may alter mood or thinking.

4. **Monitor the risk of self harm.** Promptly refer patients whom you judge should receive immediate specialist mental health services.

Approaches to treatment

There are three main ways to treat depression: with social support, with psychological therapies of various sorts, and with antidepressant medication. They are not mutually exclusive and there is some evidence that a combination can work better than either alone. All have disadvantages as well as advantages. Some older people find it difficult to express their distress in psychological language, whilst there are others who see antidepressant medication as dangerous, potentially addictive and a camouflage for their problems. Social support and activities may not be what some depressed older people want, and they will not enjoy them. Therefore, the kinds of therapies to use need to be negotiated with each person, making early discussion of explanatory models all the more important.

Offering support to depressed patients is associated with quite high rates of symptomatic recovery, and reception staff, practice nurses and staff in care homes may have a therapeutic role as important as that of doctors. These kinds of personal relationship may restore a sense of worth that has been eroded by loss of friends and family, long-term illness and loss of abilities or opportunities. Even brief encounters with an empathic and experienced person may help the depressed individual to assimilate losses (developing compensatory mechanisms like new friendships) or to accommodate to them, by changing expectations and standards. Depression in later life can then be understood as having two possible origins. The individual may fail to assimilate the challenges that go with ageing and become depressed. Or they may fail to give up past standards that were important to them and become depressed by their failure to retain their former capacity. The conversations that occur within families, among friends or between professionals and their patients/clients will reflect these distinctions: what other things can be done to offset social losses or physical disabilities, and what are realistic goals in a changed situation?

Social support seems to work by altering the thinking and feeling of older people in positive, antidepressant ways. However, it is not usually consciously psychological but simply what people do in productive and reciprocal human relationships. Psychotherapy is different because it is deliberate, framed in terms of psychological theories, frequently conducted on a one-to-one basis outside 'normal' relationships and often intense. Psychological treatments such as those recommended by the National Service Framework for Older People (cognitive behaviour therapy, interpersonal therapy and brief focal analytic psychotherapy) are effective treatments for depressive disorder in older people but are under-used (Lebowitz et al 1997). Age should not be a barrier to referring an older person for psychological therapies, but it seems to be. In patients with dementia, a carefully thought out family intervention is associated with an improvement in mood in care-givers, and so falls within the repertoire of social care as much as the local memory clinic or community mental health trust. Finally, strengthening self-efficacy by the experience of dealing with and overcoming specific problems may be the best way to approach late life depression (Blazer 2002), but there is as yet little evidence from experimental studies to support this, and therefore this is an important area for research.

Prescribing antidepressants is a medical task, but understanding the ways in which they can help and should be used is everyone's, starting with the person concerned and including community nursing staff and the social care workforce. A treatment approach to optimise concordance with medication use requires:

○ The use of medication with low risks of adverse effects. This is very important because antidepressants can cause hypotension, increase agitation and sleeplessness and (sometimes) arrhythmias.

○ A dialogue that elicits specific concerns about medication. The fear that antidepressants will not alter the underlying disease process is realistic. Similarly anxiety about becoming dependent on antidepressants is very reasonable, given the initial assurances that antidepressants were not habit-forming and the current concern that they can be difficult to stop.

○ The inclusion of care-givers (family members, homecare workers, community nurses or care home staff) in the education and motivational programme wherever possible and appropriate (Maidment et al 2002).

The choice and use of antidepressant medication should be based on the principles shown in Box 12.4.

BOX 12.4: Recommendations for practice — acute treatment phase with antidepressants

- Older people with a major depressive episode (see Chapter 1 for a definition) should be offered treatment with an antidepressant drug.
- For mild to moderate major depressive disorder a psychological intervention can be offered as an effective alternative.
- For persistent minor depression (>4 weeks) an trial of antidepressant medication should be considered.
- Antidepressant treatment should be tailored to the individual, in terms of medication type and dosage.
- Older antidepressants (like the tricyclic group) should be avoided in patients at risk of suicide.
- In patients with major depression complicating dementia, treatment with an SSRI (selective serotonin reuptake inhibitor) like fluoxetine, or with moclobemide or venlafaxine is recommended, along with increased support to the care giver.
- In patients with co-morbidity the recommended antidepressants are SSRIs, venlafaxine, mirtazapine and nefazodone.

BOX 12.4: Recommendations for practice—acute treatment
phase with antidepressants—continued

- The use of low dosages of antidepressants in major depression is
  not recommended.
- In frail patients it is advisable to 'start low, go slow' with antidepressant medication—use a low dose initially to ensure that the
  individual does not experience harmful adverse effects, and slowly
  increase it to the effective therapeutic dose.

How should treatments be tailored to individuals? To some
extent this depends on their personal history, other medical
problems and their preferences, but the nature and depth of the
depression also matters. An approach to deciding on treatment
options for the different types of depressive disorder has been
developed by the Royal College of Psychiatrists Faculty of Old
Age Psychiatry (Royal College of Psychiatrists 2002), and is
shown in Table 12.1. Tailoring can be a major of informed
judgement rather than a strict science for there is no evidence
that one antidepressant is more effective than another. The
choice of medication will be determined by patient characteristics such as:

- severity of depression—favouring tricyclics
- safety—broadly favouring newer antidepressants, except
  paroxetine
- prior response to a particular medication
- tolerability
- anticipated side-effects
- drug interactions

Table 12.1: Treatment modality and type of depression

Type of depression	Treatment modality
Psychotic depression	Combined antidepressant or ECT—urgent referral indicated
Severe/major (non-psychotic) depression	Combined antidepressant and psychological therapy—consider referral
Mild to moderate depressive episode	Antidepressant or psychological therapy (CBT, problem-solving, IPT or brief psychodynamic psychotherapy)
Dysthymia	Antidepressant
Recent onset sub-threshold (minor) depression	Watchful waiting and support
Persistent sub-threshold (minor) depression	Antidepressant and support
Brief depression, grief reaction and bereavement symptoms	Treat as for moderate depression if duration and intensity suggest intervention is indicated; otherwise support and watchful waiting
Persistent minor depression with comorbidity	Some evidence of the effectiveness of counselling

○ concordance—to what extent does the individual understand their problem, accommodate to the diagnosis and its treatment, and assimilate the therapy into everyday routines?

○ frailty

○ local protocols.

Newer antidepressants, like the SSRIs, are better tolerated than older drugs (like the tricyclics) but the difference is not great (Anderson et al 2000), and there are risks in using paroxetine (see below).

Maintenance therapy

How long should antidepressant treatments continue? The best evidence on continuation and maintenance treatment regimes, as summarised by the Royal College of Psychiatrists, suggests that:

○ maintenance therapy of 12 months for a first major depressive episode, and longer for a recurrent disorder, would be appropriate, but also that there is less certainty about treatment for non-major depression

○ nortriptyline, dosulepin (dothiepin), and citalopram can prevent recurrence

○ there is a lack of consensus on how long maintenance treatment should last or whether it should last for life.

These rules are imprecise, and decisions need to be made on a person-by-person basis. The scientific evidence also changes; for example, paroxetine is no longer an antidepressant that would be offered to older people with depression, because of the risks of dependency and adverse effects.

Given this overview of depression in later life, what would be the best approach to helping Mrs. DD on page 213?

References

Alexopoulos GS, Katz IR, Reynolds CF, Carpenter D, Docherty JP. The expert consensus guideline series: Pharmacotherapy of Depressive Disorders in Older Patients *Postgrad Med Special Report*. (October):1–86, Minneapolis: Expert Knowledge Systems, LLC, McGraw-Hill Healthcare Information Programs; 2001.

Anderson, IM, Nutt, DJ, Deakin, JFW. Evidence-based guidelines for treating depressive disorders with antidepressants: a revision of the 1993 British Association for Psychopharmacology guidelines. J Psychopharmacol 2000;14(1):3–20.

Aromaa A, Raitasalo R, Reunanen et al. Depression and cardiovascular disease. Acta Psychiatr Scand 1994; 377:77–82.

Beekman ATF, Deeg DJH, Smit JH, Vantilburg W. Predicting the course of depression in the older population — results from a community-based study in the Netherlands. J Affective Disorders 1995; 34(1):41–49.

Blazer DG. Self-efficacy and depression in late life: a primary prevention proposal. Aging and Mental Health 2002; 6:315–324.

Cole MG, Bellavance F, Mansour A. Prognosis of depression in elderly community and primary care populations: A systematic review and meta-analysis. Am J Psychiatr 1999; 156(8):1182–1189.

Eustace A, Denihan A, Bruce I, Cunningham C, Coakley D, Lawlor BA. Depression in the community-dwelling elderly: do clinical and sociodemographic factors influence referral to psychiatry? Int J Ger Psychiatr 2001; 16(10):975–979.

Lebowitz, BD, Pearson, JL, Schneider, L et al. Diagnosis and treatment of depression in late life. JAMA 1997; 278: 1186–1190.

MacDonald AJD. Do general practitioners miss depression in elderly patients? BMJ 1986; 292:1365–1367.

Maidment R, Livingston G, Katona C. 'Just keep taking the tablets': adherence to antidepressant treatment in older people in primary care. Int J Ger Psychiatr 2002; 17(8):752–757.

Ormel J, Rijsdijk FV, Sullivan M, van Sonderen E, Kempen GIJM. Temporal and reciprocal relationship between IADL/ADL disability and depressive symptoms in late life. Gerontology 2002; 57(4):338–347.

Royal College of Psychiatrists. Guideline For The Assessment And Management Of Later Life Depression In Primary Care, 2002.

Silverstone PH. Depression increases mortality and morbidity in acute life-threatening medical illness. J Psychosom Res 1990; 34:651–657.

World Psychiatric Association (WPA). WPA International Committee for Prevention and Treatment of Depression: depressive disorders in older persons. New York: NCM Publishers; 1999.

Appendices

Appendix 1 Useful addresses and telephone numbers

1. The Alzheimer's Society
Gordon House
10 Greencoat Place
London SW1P 1PH
Helpline: 0845 300 0336
General information: 020 7306 0606
http://www.alzheimers.org.uk

2. Age Concern England
Astral House
1268 London Road
London SW16 3ER
Tel No: 020 8679 8000
http://www.ageconcern.org.uk

3. MIND (National Association for Mental Health)
25–19 Broadway
Stratford
London E15 4BQ
Tel No: 020 8519 2122
http://www.mind.org.uk

4. Carers National Association
20/25 Glasshouse Yard
London EC14A 4JS
Tel No: 020 7490 8818
http://www.carersuk.demon.co.uk

5. Association of Crossroads Care Attendant Schemes
10 Regent Place
Rugby
Warwickshire CV21 2PN
Tel No: 01788 573653
Provides paid care attendants to family carers
http://www.crossroads.org.uk/

6. Counsel and Care
Twyman House
16 Bonney Street
London NW1 9PG
Tel No: 020 7485 1566
http://www.counselandcare.org.uk/
Provides list of nursing homes which they select and regularly inspect

7. Grace
35 Walnut Tree Close
Guildford
Surrey GU1 4UL
Tel No: 01483 304354
Lists private homes suitable for people with Alzheimer's disease; these are visited and assessed annually

Appendix 2 Abbreviated Mental Test (AMT)

- Age
- Time (to nearest hour)
- Address for recall (42 West Street, Gateshead)
- Year
- Where do you live (town or road)
- Recognition of two persons
- Date of birth (day and month)
- Year of start of First World War
- Name of Monarch/Prime Minister
- Count backwards 20–1

Total Score ten (one for each item)

Appendix 3 Webster's Parkinson's Disease Rating Scale (PDRS)

Enter an "x" in the appropriate column for each finding (give only 1 answer per row)			
Score	**0**	**1**	**2**	**3**
Bradykinesia of the hands				
	None	Some slowing	Moderate slowing	Severe slowing
Rigidity				
	None	Focal and mild	Moderate	Severe
Posture				
	Normal	Head starting to flex forward	Head and arms moderately flexed	Simian posture
Upper extremity swing				
	Normal	Decrease in arm swing	One arm fails to swing	Both arms fail to swing
Gait				
	Normal	Mild shortening, turns slowly	Stride moderately shortened	Shuffling gait, turns very slowly
Tremor				
	None	Mild	Not constant, some control	Constant and severe

Facies				
	Normal	Some immobility	Moderate immobility	Frozen face, severe drooling
Seborrhoea				
	No increase or change in consistency	Increased perspiration but thin	Secretions increased, thick and oily	Marked with thick secretions
Speech				
	Clear, easily understood	Slight hoarseness, loss of resonance	Monotone, dysarthria, hesitant	Very difficult to hear or understand
Self care				
	No impairment	Full self-care but rate slowed	Requires some help and slow to complete	Unable to care for self
Score				
Total score out if 30				
	1–10 = mild disability 11–20 = moderate disability 21–30 severe disability			

Reference: Webster DD. Critical analysis of the disability in Parkinson's disease. Modern Treatment 1968 ; 257–282

Index

Page numbers in *italics* refer to tables and boxes.